THE CHILD HEART

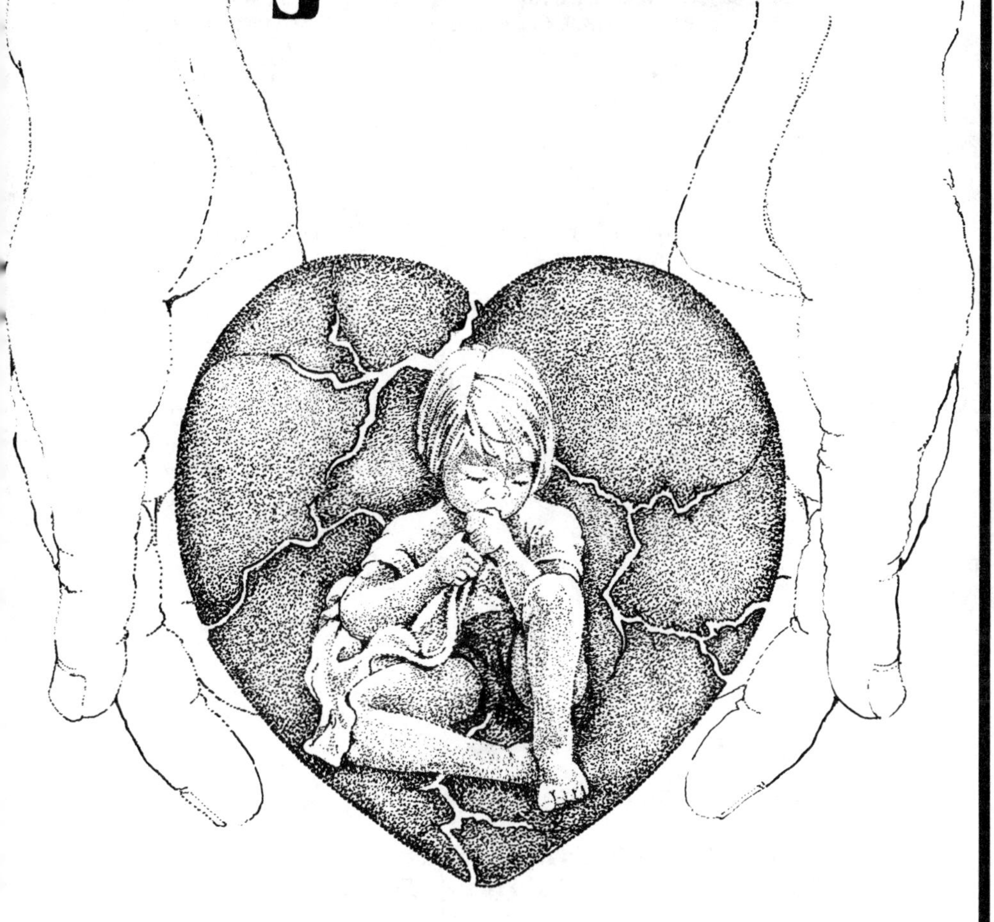

LOUIS and CAROL GORDON
KATHRYN BUTLER TURNER

FOREWORD BY GAVIN AND PATTI MacLEOD

THE CHILD HEART
ISBN 0-9627609-0-0

P.O. Box 516
Bethany, Okla. 73008-0516

Cover design by Ann Donily.

Printed in the United States of America.
1st Printing, October 1990. 2nd Printing, December 1992

CONTENTS

FOREWORD

We have known Louis and Carol Gordon for many years -- in that period of time, they have helped thousands of people. Their child heart ministry should be utilized by everyone -- as most everyone has a wounded child within him. Our bodies may mature physically, but we always have that heart of a child. The Gordons address this subject in their new book, "The Child Heart". It is pulsating with information to help us all be the free children our Father wants us to be. They instruct us how to deal with our defense mechanisms, patterns of fears, stress, counterfeit "safe areas", the pain of the wounded child heart, and the work of the Holy Spirit toward healing. They also address forgiveness and repentance -- how to pray for hurting family members and finally how we can have a whole complete life -- and who doesn't want that!! It is a book you won't be able to stop reading. Louis and Carol are an inspiration to us -- their book "The Child Heart" will be an inspiration to you.

Gavin and Patti MacLeod

INTRODUCTION

For several years after the restoration of our marriage, people had sought us out to pray for their broken relationships. We found we were teaching more and more to each one as we went along. It seemed more efficient to teach a group of people and then pray individually for specific needs. At the time of this writing, we have been ministering in classes this way for five years.

The Father has required much growth, and the laying down of our self-lives as He has taught us how to reach His people.

In 1987, He led us to begin giving "mommy and daddy hugs" to people. We receive them with the unconditional love of Jesus and give them a blessing. We also repent to them on behalf of their parents specifically, and also for others who have wounded them. We ask that they respond with forgiveness. For many, this hug seems to be the first time they have really been able to experience unconditional love. The reality of God's love drops from their head to their heart. Then they are able to receive healing from the Lord in specific areas which He reveals to them as we pray. By speaking to specific oppressions, those chains are broken and cast out by speaking in the name of Jesus. As these strongholds come down, the believers are able to walk free. They are able, if they will, to remain free by continuing to grow in their relationship to the Lord.

"The Spirit of the Sovereign Lord is on me, because the Lord has anointed me to preach the good news to the poor. He has sent me to bind up the brokenhearted, to proclaim freedom for the captives and release from darkness for the prisoners, to proclaim the year of the Lord's favor and the day of vengeance of our God, to comfort all who mourn, and provide for those who grieve in Zion -- to bestow on them a crown of beauty instead of ashes, the oil of gladness instead of mourning, and a garment of praise instead of a spirit of despair. They will be called oaks of righteousness, a planting of the Lord for the display of his splendor." (Isa. 61:1-3 NIV)

This book has come out of many hours of prayer and ministry to thousands over the last seven years, and is an attempt to share the light the Lord has given us in this needed area of healing for His body. We saw the need for healing of the hurting little child whom we heard crying inside those who had difficulty receiving the ordinary way of ministering. We had hearts which wanted to help as we had been helped. (I Cor. 1:4) We began crying out to God until He showed us how He saw His hurting children. Then He began to teach us how to minister to their needs so that He could set them free from the bondage that enslaved them. We have a growing tape ministry which deals in greater detail with specific areas.

Our vision is to plant heart mending in churches who see the need of more healing for their people. So many Christians have believed that being "born again" is all there is to having a relationship with Jesus. Others think if you are "Spirit-filled", you have arrived. These are wonderful and necessary, but only the start of developing such a fellowship with the Lord that we truly walk with Him. He wants the freedom to transform us into His image. Continual growth should be expected.

Our class is available on videotape to churches with corresponding classbooks and other teaching aids. We are happy to train pastoral and leadership couples to minister more thoroughly using these helps.

What we believe the Lord is saying is that the church is called to be balanced. On the one hand it is to be a hospital and on the other a war camp. To get people healed so that they are prepared to enter into battle is the call of Heart Menders.

A couple of notes.

First, while the examples are factual, they are modified so that identities remain confidential.

Secondly, though many of our adult responses to sin are caused by the hurts of childhood, we recognize that there are also betrayals and hurts as adults. We are not intending to ignore the carnal responses which open the door to sin.

Thirdly, this book is not intended to be a scholarly treatise on justification, sanctification, or the effects of the inherited sin nature of Adam. Rather, we want to portray the practical ramifications of these spiritual truths on individual lives and the responses we make to sin.

We appreciate the encouragement of all of the dear friends who by their prayers and lives have made this book possible. A special thanks to Darrell Smith for his help in typing.

Blessings on you all,

Louis and Carol

Louis and Carol Gordon

THE NEED FOR WHOLENESS

CHAPTER 1

"May God Himself, the God of peace, sanctify you through and through. May your whole spirit, soul, and body be kept blameless at the coming of our Lord Jesus Christ. The one who calls you is faithful and he will do it." (I Thes. 5:23-24 NIV)

What a wonderful promise! Why then are the lives of so many believers like a roller coaster ride? Why do we so often "lose it" and then feel so ashamed of our mistakes? Why do some habits and compulsions still plague us several years after accepting the Lord? Are we striving hard for approval and success, but never reaching our goal? If we have despaired of overcoming in these and other areas, what are we to do? We hear the Word preached and have excellent teaching, but are these areas of personal need ever really addressed?

Until we really begin to receive the light of the Word on our problems, it is hard to understand ourselves. Life is such a see-saw, rocking back and forth, back and forth. Stability and consistency are pipe dreams. The enormity of the frustration is tremendous, especially for Christians. After all, if we are supposed to be new creatures in Christ Jesus, why the chronic problems, the constant struggles? Why is it the same old issues arise over and over?

Where is total, complete and long-lasting victory? Why does peace flit in and out of our lives, never stopping, only teasing us with its promise? Where is the rest of God for our emotions?

Anguish shadows us. Insecurity and fear freely ride slipshod over our minds even while we are in the midst of trying to pray. We end up denying our innermost pain instead of finding healing. Driven by rejection and fear we habitually wrestle with torment in almost every relationship, whether it be our parents, spouse, children, friends or co-workers.

Our emotions have evolved under the influence of a wounded, scarred child heart. Abnormality is seen as real life; also,

Success	versus	Failure
Joy	versus	Frustration
Freedom	versus	Slavery (Self-consciousness)
Winning	versus	Losing, and even
Life	versus	Death.

All of these are child heart issues. The fractured wounded child has ruled our lives. When we do not experience deep, intense, unconditional, and protective love from our parents, then a door opens for fear and then rejection. The little child heart knows something is wrong. One side of the soul gets stunted as that fear pours in. That part of the heart does not seem to mature as the rest of the person develops. The other part grows up normally. No matter what opened the door to it's wounding, the child heart needs healing. It is very rare to find anyone who doesn't have some type of hurt in their heart. It is so common, that most of us suffer from a defensive, wounded child heart.

The influence of this pain which usually starts early in life has far-reaching tentacles. Instead of walking as conquerors, we are conquered. We, who should be victors, behave as victims. Rather than acting as children of the King, we carry ourselves as step-children of paupers. It is as if we can't help ourselves. Our wounds influence our decisions, personal relationships, and business dealings. There is no question that most of us are not triumphing in the victory that is promised to us as Christians, which causes more problems.

Discouragement has caused the downfall of more than one believer. We must recognize and deal with, by the Holy Spirit, all the old covered up hurts and traumas. The fact that sometimes the source of pain is not easily recalled is not a problem to the Holy Spirit. He will bring to light only what in His wisdom He knows we are ready to handle.

The hurt of the wounded child heart not only shapes our own lives from childhood, but also those around us.

Since most people encounter deep pain and rejection before the age of six, the world has been buffeted by the effects of these wounds. We meet and have to deal with wounded people every day of our lives. It is a serious issue. But, THERE IS HOPE! People everywhere are responding to this life-giving revelation. Louis and Carol shared about the wounded child heart for only ten minutes at a meeting of 800 people where they had been invited to share. When it was time for the altar call, Louis said, "I want everyone to stand up that....."

The Lord stopped him for a second as 600 people stood.

"Wait!" he said, "You don't even know what I'm going to say. I'm wanting all those who suffer from a defensive, wounded child's heart to stand and continue to stand." More people joined the 600 already standing. Not one took a seat.

Louis and Carol ministered corporately to those standing. For the next several days, people kept coming up to them saying, "Now I know what's been causing me to act the way I have." And, "We now understand what's going on with our relationships... wife... husband... kids... or friends."

Later, the Lord led them to give Momma's and Daddy's hugs of healing and blessing. When they did this, many people just broke down and sobbed. They had been so thirsty for love. Their wounded little child hearts had been starved for a healing touch.

Our child hearts need healing.

Once we begin to allow the work of the Holy Spirit in our lives, we will be able to experience victory in Christ. Instead of a habitual struggle, our lives begin to smooth out into more peace and joy, caring and acceptance, healing and fulfillment. This process will change the dynamics of our families as well as in our own personal lives.

As the following chapters shed light into previously hidden corners of the heart, please grasp the realities of what is being shared for yourself.

It was asked how Jesus learned the things He taught. His answer was (John 7:16 NIV), **"My teaching is not my own. It comes from him who sent me. If anyone chooses to do God's will, he will find out whether my teaching comes from God or whether I speak on my own."** We ask that you apply the same test to this book. Let the Lord confirm to you His truth.

To those who believed Him, Jesus said (John 8:31-32 NIV), **"If you hold to my teaching, you are really my disciples. Then you will know the truth, and the truth will set you free."**

THE WOUNDING OF THE CHILD HEART

CHAPTER 2

What is important to God is also important to the devil. In Jeremiah 1:5, the Lord says that He knew us even in the womb. God has known us since conception. If God loves us enough to be intimately aware of us from our beginnings, it follows that satan attempts to know us that early as well. He tries to begin his destructive patterns as early as possible.

One reason why the enemy attacks so hard in our child's heart is so that, even at a very early age, we won't be able to recognize the faithfulness of the love of Jesus. The earlier the enemy can block this knowledge, the more difficult it is for us to learn of the grace, mercy and blessings of the Lord. There will be that much extra time for rejection, fear, and of course, hurtful memories. The agony compounds as we grow older. The consequence is a cancerous double-mindedness that grows with every life crisis with a disastrous result. We become more and more confused as to whom to turn to in times of trouble. Our needs aren't being met, and the confusion feeds on the emotional chaos.

Many Christians suffer from double-mindedness. We do not even begin to realize how destructive it can be. Part of our being wants to draw closer to Jesus, and the other part is afraid He will fail us or require more than we can yield. It appears to us that when the child heart is wounded by both a lack of nurture and by a lack of hugs and prayers of parents, the soul shatters. There are far too many people in the Body of Christ who are double-minded. It eats away at every Christian who suffers from it. On one hand, there is a heart which wants to draw closer to Jesus, while on the other, there's a lot of junk which is weighing it down, slowing it down, and tripping up the Christian walk.

"If any of you lacks wisdom, he should ask God, who gives generously to all without finding fault, and it will be given him. But when he asks, he must believe and not doubt, because he who doubts is like a wave of the sea, blown and tossed by the wind. That man should not think he will receive anything from the Lord; he is a double-minded man, unstable in all he does." (James 1:5-8 NIV)

God knows the importance of our being single-minded. He wants us to be that way, and He intends it so that we can be stable in all of our ways. This stability is essential if we expect to receive everything we need from Him. When we are single-minded, we recognize Him as our source in every area: spiritually, physically, emotionally, financially, socially; in every aspect of life.

As we found ourselves ministering to numbers of hurting people several years ago, we began to cry out to the Lord for a key to their healing. After hundreds of hours of prayer we received an answer. One night, the Lord spoke to Louis and said, "I never intended my children to have **a spirit of fear, but one of power, love and a sound mind."** (2 Tim 1:7) The Lord went on to say, "But the devil perpetrates fear on the little child heart at a very early age, sometimes even in the mother's womb. Instead of the power that I intended, the devil brings in fear, helplessness, hopelessness, and selfishness. Instead of the love that I intended, the devil brings in rejection, rebellion, and betrayal. Instead of the sound mind that I intended, the devil brings in the double-mindedness, a split personality, and schizophrenia."

What revelation! How we rejoice in the fact that there is hope and help for the hurting, that there is a reason behind the confusion.

It makes sense. Satan destroys. He is not a creator. Because he himself is a created entity, it has always been impossible for him to create anything. Therefore, he is a perverter. If he can, he will always grab at what God has created and purposed for good, and will pervert it in some manner, destroying it if possible.

He hammers away at people, even while in the womb. With the tools of rejecting words, strife between parents, and thoughts of abortion, satan will cause a fracturing in the child's heart. This fragmenting of the soul is certainly evident in double-mindedness, at the very least; that is to be torn by wanting to follow Jesus and by wanting to follow the flesh. The enemy's purpose is the death and destruction of God's goodness and creation. To do this, satan strives to cut us off from the love of the Lord so that these perversions can grow like a wildfire in a gale out of control.

One major ploy of the enemy is to cut off the headship of the home. Satan wants the family out of balance, so he tries to shut down the father image in people's lives. He also negates the value of the mother and her role as well whenever possible.

By taking the father out of the home, the father's spiritual covering is compromised. Death, illness, divorce, and war all keep a father away from his children. Other things can, too. Workaholism, alcoholism, and excessive hobbies show the child that he is less important than whatever else is going on in his daddy's life. When that happens the child heart begins to fracture. There is also a type of father who does not function as a godly father, even when he is home. A father who is abusive when drunk, abusive when sober, or full of hate, pity, and guilt, is not functioning as a father, but plays more of a child's role. He wants to be taken care <u>of</u> instead of caring <u>for</u> his children. His own wounded child heart demands precedence over his own family and their needs. His pain sets up a cycle of even more pain for his children and his children's children.

Many daddies don't have these types of debilitating problems, but, a lot of fathers were not raised in a nurturing environment. Their fathering can be less than effective, thereby perpetuating the wounded child's heart to their own children. Rejection will always beget rejection.

Besides providing a spiritual covering, the earthly father is our natural example of what the Heavenly Father is like. By cutting us off from our earthly father's love, we quickly learn to have little ability to believe that God would really love us. The relationship with the earthly father plays a critical role in how we relate to our Heavenly Father. There is usually a direct correlation. If the earthly relationship is hindered, then the child will have trouble trusting in and relating to the Lord. God uses the father/child relationship as the point of reference for building a relationship with Him, the Heavenly Father. Children need the paternal covering.

Another hindrance in the development of a healthy child heart is an unhealthy relationship between the mother and father. How a mother and father treat one another, even how they view each other, can affect their children's little child hearts. Men are to love their wives, and wives are to respect and honor their husbands. If the father doesn't really protect the mother tenderly, or if the mother doesn't hold the father in high regard, the family is spiritually dysfunctional. It is out of scriptural order. (Eph. 5:21-33) The parents' disobedience in their marital relationship creates a chink in the covering of God's perfect family plan. The covering is not as complete as the Lord intended, thereby leaving an open door for the enemy to score wounds against every member. Children in particular are jeopardized. Not able to develop in the healthiest possible manner, their emotional and spiritual health are compromised.

"Jack" and "Doris" couldn't stand each other the first twenty years of marriage. Neither one of them walked in a godly manner in their marriage. Doris despised Jack and spoke badly of him to others, and, when she felt like it, to his face as well. To escape from her, Jack stayed away from home as much as possible. He didn't like being around her. Any place was more peaceful than home. Their attitudes towards each other wounded the hearts of all of their children. Because they did not nurture one another in the Lord, they could not provide necessary nurturing to their kids. As their children grew up, their behaviors were chaotic and full of rebellion.

After Doris and Jack met Jesus, He changed their hearts. They became tender toward each other. They learned to love each other. Eventually, Jack and Doris felt that they needed to repent to their children for the hatred which had been displayed in their marriage relationship for so long. As Jack and Doris established a new, caring relationship with each other, they were able to establish new, caring relationships with their children. Although now adults, the children in turn became kinder and more responsible, and a healing of their child hearts began.

Is a godly marriage easy to accomplish? Of course not, as many of us can certainly testify. Since most marriage partners themselves have wounded child hearts, scriptural adherence to loving the wife and honoring the husband is almost impossible. It requires a continual laying down of the self-life. It requires a walk of constant forgiveness. It requires the reign of Jesus in our hearts, especially concerning a spouse who doesn't even come close to

Christian behavior. In marriage, there needs to be a godly reaction to ungodly action. That's really hard to do.

For instance, perhaps the father is an alcoholic, hitting the bars every night, and neglecting his family. The mother still must honor his role as head of the household. She may not honor, love, or respect his alcoholic behavior, but she must honor, love, and respect him. This is not an easy task, especially when there are children involved, but it is scriptural. She can pray I Timothy 3:2-8 over him. Children must also be taught this same principle of honoring and praying for the head of the household. (See Eph. 6:2-3)

Sometimes of course, it is the mother who is out of order, insisting on taking over the spiritual headship of the home, controlling the home, insisting on having her way, and dominating every situation. Then, the father must continue to love her and cherish her, while praying Scriptures such as Proverbs 31 over her. No matter what the problem, each spouse should recognize and intercede on behalf of the other one's need for healing.

When godly responses to ungodly behaviors take place, the children grow up in a more healthy manner. If natural (sinful) reactions to ungodly behaviors occur, then everyone suffers, no one wins. The child heart of every member of the family is stunted. Continuing with the example of the disease of alcoholism, instead of condemning the alcoholic, recognize the destructive behavior for the horribleness it is. However, begin to respect and cherish the hurting person inside. When the alcoholic is judged and condemned, bitterness sets in, and the children will be more apt to become alcoholics themselves. In the situation of a bossy, dominating mother, if she is condemned and judged, the children will become more like her, reflecting the controlling behavior in their own lives. Acceptance of the spouse is paramount in the prevention of wounding the child heart in the lives of the children. Forgiveness helps to loosen those deadly chains of generational behaviors, with the result that the children have a better opportunity for solid emotional health.

Both poor marriage relationship and the taking of the parents out of the home through one means or another injures and paralyzes the child heart.

Satan goes after the families so that he can destroy successive generations. God's plan was for healthy children. (Mal. 2:15 AMP) **"And did not God make you and your wife one flesh? Did not One make you and preserve your spirit alive? And why did God make you two one? Because He sought a godly offspring [from your union]. Therefore, take heed to yourselves, and let no one deal treacherously and be faithless to the wife of his youth."**

Look at the tactics the devil uses. It is horrifying to see not only the effect he has had in our own lives, but what is happening in everyone else's life as well. His destruction is becoming pervasively acceptable throughout the entire world with very few voices raised with the truth of what is going on.

A very visible weapon the devil uses in this destruction is the death of the child. In ancient times plagues and diseases took the lives of thousands of children before they even had much of a chance of living. Whole families would be wiped out. Not only the child, but also the mother and father died at the hands of these widespread epidemics.

Innocents were slaughtered on the altars of perversion during pagan ceremonial rites. **"Do not give any of your children to be sacrificed to Molech, for you must not profane the name of your God. I am the LORD."** (Lev. 18:21 NIV) Countless children were butchered; infanticide in the name of false gods. The killing was supposed to ensure a better life for everyone else. Prosperity was the promise for killing the babies. This type of worship was prevalent in many of the ancient cultures.

Satan still uses the tactic of death today. Abortion now takes over where child sacrifice left off. The enemy wants to destroy the child before his birth so that not only his life and future are eradicated, but the matter is complicated by involving the mother and doctor in the murderous sin. This open door of complicity allows even more perversion and sin to hammer at them for the rest of their lives.

To Christians, abortion is a very obvious maneuver of destruction. Most Christian parents do not participate in the practice. It's not an option. If they ever have experienced abortion in the past, many have sought and received forgiveness. But Christians can sometimes be influenced by subliminal, societal messages. No less dangerous and much more devious than abortion is the manner of how children are really viewed and treated in our culture.

Through the changing of the proper loving attitude that parents are supposed to have towards their young, a wounded child heart quickly develops in a young child. We need only to look around us. This is exactly what is happening in today's culture. With rare exceptions, children are considered inconvenient, troublesome, and expensive; a stumbling block to a standard of living that couples believe is a necessity of life to which they are entitled. Most of our "necessities" aren't. Nonetheless, they and their acquisition push children out of the way.

There is an all-encompassing thought pattern towards today's kids. It is definitely not pro-child. In fact, presently there is a push to get children out of the home and into school at the age of four, so that life will be more convenient for the parents. The baby wants to be with his mommy, not a public school teacher or a "child care professional". Satan is moving to destroy the home base by using an anti-child attitude in our culture. We are ultimately selling our children for a nicer house, car and clothes. Of course, this is not to cause confusion for the single working mother, or any other mother, who has to work just to get food on the table. But, for the majority of families, children get in the way of the almighty dollar, and are farmed out. "Self-fulfillment" should not be an altar on which to sacrifice children. As the children get older, their needs are bought off with material things so that mom and dad won't have to put any time investment into them.

It was God's intent that a child be physically fed and nurtured at it's mother's breast. The devil, and our culture, have conspired to make it easy for mothers to choose not to nurse their babies. This needs to be a matter of serious prayer for parents-to-be. This is in fact one of the indications that confirm that we are in the end times. Jesus said, "**Daughters of Jerusalem, do not weep for me; weep for yourselves and for your children. For the time will come when you will say, 'Blessed are the barren women, the wombs that never bore and the breasts which never nursed.' Then they will say to the mountains, 'Fall on us!' and to the hills, 'Cover us.' For if men do these things when the tree is green, what will happen when it is dry?**" (Luke 23:28-31 NIV)

All these attitudes cause a wounded child's heart in young children which they carry with them as they mature into adulthood. That learned behavior is then passed onto their children, and the cycle continues.

We heard a story recently about snow geese. They mate for life, and never desert their offspring. It is reported that a whole flock of geese had laid eggs and were sitting on the nest, when an untimely snowstorm began. As the snow piled higher and higher, they would <u>not</u> leave the eggs, even for a breath of air. They were found later, stretching their necks upward to try to get their last breath. They died of suffocation, never leaving their commitment to each other and their offspring. How many of today's parents are willing to make that kind of commitment? How many parents realize what level of love is required to bring about that type of commitment?

When the child heart senses it is unwanted, even in the womb, it begins to wither from the rejection. Not only negative attitudes, but also negative words towards the unborn, and very young, damage the child heart. Verbal abuse is just as deadly as physical abuse. These words and attitudes don't have to come from a parent, either. When there is inadequate prayer cover, someone else's words and attitudes can harm the young child.

"Lori's" mother faced the news of her unexpected pregnancy with a happy sort of trepidation. Nervous, because it would be her third child in three years, and money was tight. Nervous, because she had had difficult labors with her other two babies. But, very joyful because she recognized babies as a direct blessing from the Lord.

Little Lori's grandmother was not so delighted. In fact, she was extremely upset. She encouraged an abortion the first couple of weeks after she first found out about the upcoming arrival. The parents ignored her. Then, the encouraging hints and suggestions about an abortion evolved into an urging. Grandmother began insisting. She warned Lori's mother that it would be too hard to have another child right now. The last one was still in diapers. There would be too much work. Where would the money come from? What about the other two? They wouldn't get enough attention. They would absolutely hate their new brother or sister. Things would just be awful, and no one would want to babysit three little ones. The whole situation would be impossible with another baby. The parents were irresponsible, and stupid to be having another child.

On and on she harangued the family. Lori's daddy finally asked her not to speak of the matter again. She was told to drop it.

Baby Lori was born on a lovely spring day. She was beautiful and healthy, but with no apparent reason, cried non-stop the first twelve months of her life. The poor baby was always upset. Although they did everything they knew to do, Lori's mother and father were at their wits' end. Nothing seemed to make Lori peaceful and happy. It was hard on the entire family.

When Lori was three years old, her mother and father learned about the child heart and received healing for their own wounded child hearts. As they were healed, the Holy Spirit revealed to them that little Lori also had a wounded child heart; crippled from the time in the womb when her grandmother wanted her aborted. Wounded by those negative, rejecting words and attitudes that went unchallenged by her parents during their prayer time before her birth, those words and attitudes stunted Lori's little child heart before she was born, and she cried out as a baby in an emotional pain.

Lori's parents interceded for their little girl. They came against the powers of darkness which had chained Lori to unhappiness. They broke the curses of death and rejection, pain and unhappiness. They pronounced healing as they asked the Lord to fill her hurt places with peace and acceptance. They proclaimed her wanted and desired, cherished and loved.

Such a metamorphosis took place! Her entire personality changed. Lori began to smile more than she cried. She started laughing instead of sobbing. Several years later, her little heart is whole and at peace with the unconditional love of her heavenly Father. This change of happiness continues to this day. Her teachers have remarked on many occasions over her bubbly personality and her already deep faith.

Words and attitudes damage the young and affect them all of their lives. During intercession, the Holy Spirit revealed to "Margaret" and a friend that a deep rejection had taken place towards Margaret before her birth. Many words had been spoken about her while she was still in her mother's womb; hurtful words and statements of such rejection that they affected her for years. When she received healing for her wounded child's heart, her entire life and marriage changed. Seeing the difference in Margaret's life, her husband was open to having his child heart healed. Their marriage is growing and happy today.

Another weapon satan uses to destroy the child heart is an absence of touch. As discussed earlier, a wounded child heart develops in the young child by not receiving enough nurturing. Being hugged, loved, and prayed for by mom and dad is essential in growing up healthy. Love manifesting as hugs and cuddles provides security for the young child. Physical nurturing is really God revealing His Father heart. It is His nature that He wants us to be hugged, loved, and cared for. When that physical caring is not there, the door is open to fear, rejection, and the rest of the garbage that satan tries to put on us. We grow up with all of that shadowing our lives.

Most of us are familiar with what happened at a hospital in London during World War II. Babies, in the nursery, were well fed and kept disease free. But, every few days a child died for no apparent reason. Finally, it was discovered that the lack of holding, caressing, and rocking was killing the children. Cuddling our children is that important. It gives life.

So much depends on our foundational years and the relationship within the family. If a child was truly nurtured by his parents, then he would want to be just like daddy and mommy. Genuine unconditional love is a shield of armor against the attacks on the child heart. This type of active love teaches more about God's character than any other action which a parent does, because unconditional love is the type of love God has towards us.

"I love you."

No strings attached.

"I love you."

Even when you make mistakes. Even when you sin.

"I love you."

No matter how you look. No matter how I feel.

"I love you."

Unconditional love. Would we be the same people today if we had been raised with that type of love? What would our relationship with God be like if we had seen the love of the Heavenly Father in our own parents?

If this type of information rings a bell in our hearts, we can take courage that Jesus has the answers! He is more than able to restore our hearts to wholeness!

No matter how precious our parents are to us, none of them have been perfect, and of course neither are we. But God can do much for the person who will allow Jesus to heal his heart.

Let us examine our hearts. Let's go to God in prayer and ask Him to reveal how we have been hurt. Perhaps it was a parent's suicide. Maybe it was a deep loneliness because no one was ever home, loving and nurturing the little child we once were. Whether it was a divorce, death, or society's attitude towards children in general, we probably will discover that our hearts have been wounded. Whatever has happened, we can face it with the Lord's help so that it can be overcome and healed. If there are still questions whether the child heart has been hurt, look at the behaviors and attitudes experienced in life. They are excellent barometers of deep, hidden hurts.

"Now I rejoice, not because you were pained, but because the pain led you to turn back to God. For you handled the pain in God's way, so that you were not harmed by us at all. Pain handled in God's way produces a turning from sin to God which leads to salvation, and there is nothing to regret in that! But pain handled in the world's way produces only death." (II Cor. 7:9,10 JNT)

THE PAIN OF THE WOUNDED CHILD HEART

CHAPTER 3

"Jess" flung the front door open. Everyone looked up from what they were doing. Daddy was home.

"You darn dog! Get out of my way!" It yelped as it tried to avoid Jess's foot.

Loosening his tie, he jerked the refrigerator door open looking for something cold to help cool his temper down as well as counteract his hot drive home.

"Hello, Jess." His wife braved the kitchen. "Big day at the office?"

"Big day? Try bad day, a VERY bad day." He took a deep swig from his soft drink. "My secretary took off early leaving me with a lot of unfinished work which made three different customers hopping mad. Then the boss came down wanting yesterday's report, heard all of the commotion and chewed on me up one side and down the other." Jess slammed his pop down on the table in remembered anger.

"On top of that, the air conditioner in the car went out on my way home!"

He spied his son's schoolbooks at the end of the table. "I've told Matt to keep those books out of the kitchen. "Matt!" he yelled, "Get yourself in here and get this mess cleaned up." He slammed his son's books off the table and across the kitchen.

Fearfully, Matt quickly slipped into the room and began to gather his things.

"I've told you to keep your junk in your own room and out of my way", he hollered at his son. Seeing his son's eyes fill with tears, rage went all over Jess again. "Quit feeling sorry for yourself! It's time for you to grow up and get control of your emotions." He booted the eight year old as the child ran from the room.

"Where's dinner? I work hard to support this family. The least you could do is to have dinner ready for me when I get home. I don't know why people can't do what they're supposed to do and be a little more considerate around here. My goodness. You'd think we were a bunch of heathens the way you all act. Never mind" he stormed at his wife as she began to apologize. "I just won't eat. It probably wouldn't be any good anyway." With that Jess stomped off to his room and slammed his door shut.

A few hours later, he came out. "I'm sorry. I just lost control. The pressure at work .... I don't know, something just came over me. I'll do better next time. I promise I'll keep my emotions under control. I guess I just need to pray harder about my attitudes. I don't know. I am sorry."

Jess was not living the victorious life. When the pressures of his workday overwhelmed him, he flipped out. Anger, self-pity, and accusations spilled out from him. It was poured onto anyone weaker, usually his family. Even if his boss was angry, and even if his secretary had broken her commitments to him, they weren't the problem. His reactions came from his wounded child heart. His pain came from his past, manifesting in his present, and more than likely flourishing in his future. If Jess had handled the situations from a mature, wholly healed heart, a lot of the confusion at the job could have been diffused. His day would have ended happier. So what if work had been fraught with crisis? Jess could have still brought peace home to his family, and the evening would have been salvaged. The Lord would have been glorified. His wife, son, and definitely the dog would have been happier and healthier. Jess would have felt victorious. Instead, his life patterns of anger, self-pity, and blaming the other guy caused fear in the hearts of his family, thereby perpetuating the wounding of child hearts.

Self-help books and pop psychology give lots of advice for a guy with Jess's problems. Use self-control. Think of something pleasant when pressure builds. Start hobbies. Or even ignore the problem and it will go away. It won't matter which mind tricks Jess uses on himself, his tendencies to rage and feel sorry for himself will still be carried in his heart. They can't be tricked away. Ignoring woundedness won't help either. Just because something is suppressed does not make it healed. Denial does not indicate all is well.

Those defense mechanisms come screaming from the woundedness of the child heart. Another name for these behaviors are life patterns. These feelings flare up when pressure begins to mount. A pattern emerges. An otherwise normal acting person slips into these defense mechanisms when he feels stress. It grows in seriousness. These wounds evolving into life patterns deal with the area of the soul. The soulish reaction to pain can open the door to demonic oppression that affects the spirit. This in turn reinforces these troubling behavior patterns. **"The night is nearly over; the day is almost here. So let us put aside the deeds of darkness and put on the armor of light."** (Rom. 13:12 NIV)

In all of the years of ministry, we have found only one man that has had a whole, happy child heart with no oppressions of any kind. EVERYBODY ELSE has had some type of injured child heart.

In her own life, Carol's wounded child heart displayed behaviors of distrust of feelings and a non-responsiveness to emotion. This showed up as a great reluctance to experience life. Her emotions were frozen. She was afraid to laugh, and she dreaded crying. She took no risks and made no waves in her relationships. Carol was so uptight over the process of living that she appeared very compliant in dealing with her life. She avoided confrontations at all costs and really just wanted to feel safe. That craving for emotional safety was one of the main reasons she married Louis. She thought that he would be a haven of security. He appeared very non-threatening and came across as a very stable person.

As she laughs about it now, "He sure didn't turn out to be that way at all."

Conversely, Louis' own wounded heart demanded a kind, loving mate. He was needing someone who could accept him and his pain with unconditional acceptance. He thought Carol's compliant attitude came from a secure heart, full of tenderness and love. It turned out that he was really wrong, too. Instead of love and stability, Louis and Carol brought great pain into their relationship.

Consequently, after she married Louis, Carol's emotional life grew worse. Desiring to please Louis, Carol became more and more compliant, submerging her own personality. Always insecure and frightened as a child, Carol's defense mechanisms grew stronger as her own children were born. Deeply buried anxiety and fear dominated her life to such a degree that she became extremely manipulative. This manipulation was very deceptive. She saw herself as a martyr. What people saw of Carol was not what they got. She tried to build an image of a loving family, but there was no substance. She loved her children but could not acknowledge or deal with their problems. With her own fears pursuing her, she tried to cope with the disasters and make the best of everything. Denial of any of her needs was the only way she could cope with waking up each morning to a new day full of the unknown. Carol was a wound-up spring waiting to explode. Louis was hurting so much himself, he couldn't help her. He was gone a lot from home, a workaholic, because he was so unhappy at home. He buried a lot of anger and frustration at home, and then he vented these emotions in his work. He never directly lashed out at Carol, but neither could he give Carol what she needed. He withheld his best from his family and gave his time and money to other projects. He ignored the needs of the children as a passive retaliation for his own unhappiness. Their family was made up of five individuals going in five different paths of pain as Carol tried to keep everything from falling apart; while Louis tried to stay out of the family scene altogether.

Like Jess, Carol was full of hurt which affected her family. But, her anger and pain couldn't be hidden even in good times. She had convinced herself that if she didn't take care of herself through the controlling of her environment, no one else would take care of her. She was on a one-way street to frantic despair.

Then one evening, she realized that only Jesus could take care of her, and she didn't have the ability to direct anyone's life, especially her own. She accepted Christ gratefully, and gently that all-consuming need for security eased somewhat. Still, however, she could not trust emotions. Her life's experience was that emotions were tyrannical in nature and would blow her from this way to that way. Although born again, her praise and worship of the Lord was purely by faith. There was never any spark of feeling in her heart. It was as if she was frozen. Although a Christian living in God's love, Carol still did not trust feelings. It took the healing of her child heart before she could enjoy the emotional side of her life.

"Come to me, all of you who are struggling and burdened, and I will give you rest. Take my yoke upon you and learn from me, because I am gentle and humble in

heart, and you will find rest for your souls. For my yoke is easy and my burden is light." (Matt. 11:28-30 JNT)

Some sort of fear is always seen when there is a fractured child heart. Fear is the first door opening for the rest of the ugliness the devil has put on us. Then, the enemy tries to replay all the old things that were in our souls and attempts to bind us into all of those old life patterns. Most of us are very quick to walk away from obvious sins of the flesh. We try to follow most of the Ten Commandments. But our reaction to life gives us away. The sinful responses in our hearts to things that are done to us are the ones that are hidden and difficult to deal with. It's as if we want to bury those things which we don't want to think about anymore. Yet, those old life patterns are coming back to haunt us all the time. Jess was shadowed by rage and self-pity. Carol lived with insecurity and fear.

Often, we have a hard time dealing with a particular situation that recurs from time to time and have no conscious idea why it continues to be a stress in our lives.

"Betty" had a perception that as an intelligent adult she should be able to cope with any situation. Sounds familiar doesn't it? She adjusted, made the best of, and re-evaluated, whenever the circumstances required it. She always "did the right thing" or performed whatever duty came her way. One life pattern of hers was to always keep busy (translated: never relax).

A duty she thought proper was to visit close relatives in another city. She felt like it should be done periodically. These same relatives also visited her family on a regular basis.

Whenever Betty went to visit, it would usually be pretty pleasant. At least it seemed so on the surface. However, underneath it all, the childhood memories of anxiety to please, never being good enough, and feeling like a powerless child would stir up within Betty. Those feelings she kept deeply denied. The whole process of denying them made Betty very cranky for days after her return home. She would blow up at her husband and pick at him about trivial incidents. For years, her husband believed that those relatives talked badly about him to his wife, because Betty was always so hateful to him after visiting them.

When the relatives would come to visit at Betty's house, she would be beside herself preparing for their visit, believing that the house would be "inspected" and be found wanting. When they would leave she always wondered why she had gotten into such a snit. They always assured her that they had had such a nice time.

After Betty came to know Jesus, she began to allow Him to show her the condition of her heart. Little by little, He revealed the strongholds, thought patterns in her mind and emotions, which had reinforced her fear and anxiety. She began to see family relationships more realistically. She began to deal with them according to the Word of God. Betty was able to release anger and a fear of domination. She learned to forgive, thereby repenting of judging her family. Today, she realizes that much of the perception of being judged critically was in her own fear of being criticized. The insecurity of her foundation before she stabilized her life on the Rock has all been healed in Christ Jesus.

As adults, many of us are unaware of traits that reveal a wounded child heart. Like Betty, we believe it is just "the way we are." Most of us compensate for areas that we perceive to be "weak" by developing "strengths." Some of the walls which we believe make us strong can come tumbling down in a time of added stress. How many of us return home from work wiped out, not because of the physical energy required, but because of the stress of interaction with others?

Psalm 16:6 says, **"the lines are fallen unto me in pleasant places."**

In studying the scriptural references to "lines and boundaries" we can see that there are perimeters the Lord set in our lives which we are to respect and allow Him to determine. In Deut. 27:17 the third curse pronounced on Mt. Ebal was not to **"move the boundaries"**. When we stretch out, it is to be at the discretion of the Lord. Otherwise we are rebelling against God or usurping someone else's territory.

Wounded people will try to set up counterfeit safety barriers. We will establish limited perimeters that we feel are a protection. Maybe we stay at home a lot, finding projects and hobbies to drown ourselves in. Maybe like Carol, we set up a boundary of control and inaction around our lives. Or maybe we take jobs where we can just go to work with minimum interaction with co-workers.

The stress of the one soul's pull on another's mind, will, and emotions is very difficult for some of us. We fear the interaction that takes place normally among people.

Those who plead, "Well, I'm just a nervous type person" are covering up through denying a need for healing. Often we set up a protective wall to keep us from having to interface with certain people by becoming offended at them. Offense and isolation are some of the enemy's favorite ploys! If we are hurt, we withdraw. A typical pattern is not going to church when we are having problems! If we will allow the Lord to work out relationships, it will very likely turn out to be a blessing.

There are many feelings, behaviors, and attitudes which we experience that clearly indicate a wounded child heart. Denial often plays a role, as does the justification of "well, that is just the way I am." Well, it's not the way we have to be if the child heart receives its healing. The pain and fear which controls our lives can be put to rest.

Some behaviors, attitudes, and feelings are discussed in the next chapters. They are usually pretty good indicators of a wounded child heart, and when discovered can be dealt with through God's healing power.

It takes a work of the Holy Spirit in us to reveal the deceptions of our own heart. Jer. 17:9-10 (NIV) says, **"The heart is deceitful above all things and beyond cure. Who can understand it? I the Lord search the heart and examine the mind,...."** I Cor 2:10-12 (NIV) encourages us, **"but God has revealed it to us by his Spirit. The Spirit searches all things, even the deep things of God. For who among men knows the thoughts of a man except the man's spirit within him? In the same way no one knows the thoughts of God except the Spirit of God. We have not**

received the spirit of the world but the Spirit who is from God, that we may understand what God has freely given us."

As we allow the Spirit of the Lord to bring light through our spirit to our soul, we will be able to see the deceptions the enemy has sold us. By renewing our minds with God's truth, we can be set free.

BEHAVIORS AND ATTITUDES

CHAPTER 4

By now, many of us are recognizing the pain of the fractured child heart in our own lives. For most of us, this teaching brings a great sense of relief. The unnamed pain from across the years finally has an identity. The Scriptures encourage us that no matter how long these structures of pain have been with us, God has an answer. The promise of freedom rings out from every page. Isaiah 29:19-21 (NIV) cries out with joy, **"Once more the humble will rejoice in the Lord; the needy will rejoice in the Holy One of Israel. The ruthless will vanish, the mockers will disappear, and all who have an eye for evil will be cut down--those who with a word make a man out to be guilty, who ensnare the defender in court and with false testimony deprive the innocent of justice."**

But, for others who might still have some questions if this teaching is for them, take time to examine some of the following behaviors and attitudes. Although not all of the possible manifestations of a wounded child heart are listed, these are the more common problems that tyrannize our lives.

1. FEELINGS OF INFERIORITY.

Feelings of inferiority coupled with the fear of rejection flash a neon light which points directly to a wounded child heart. These feelings are so prevalent that entire sections of bookstores are dedicated to overcoming these emotional killers. Memories of past rejection reinforces feelings of present inadequacy. A very serious problem, the sense of inferiority erupts whenever a person gets around someone he perceives as important. It could be a socially prominent citizen. It could be co-workers or former professors. Anyone who is perceived as having authority or power; people with money, people with fancy titles, even certain friends.

The pain can be incapacitating. If the esteem is not returned, the individual will sink lower, feel more inferior. The expectation of rejection due to a nebulous inadequacy feeds itself and inferiority flourishes.

"Who cares what I have to say?" "I'm not worth anything." "I'm not important enough." "Why do I even try?" "If he is interested in me and wants to talk to me, he must have ulterior motives. What does he want?"

When inferiority goes on long enough, self-pity also creeps in and melds inferiority even closer to the marrow of the soul.

Inferiority certainly plays havoc with a dating life. It's a pretty common dilemma. A girl starts liking a guy. He becomes interested. They go out. As he starts liking her more and more, she dumps him.

"After all," she reasons, "If he likes me (who is not worth very much) then there must be something wrong with him. He must not be worth much either."

How many times have we seen that scenario play out this type of thinking? How many friendships have been shot down before they've had a chance to take hold? It even contributes to abusive situations. Some beaten down souls can not get out of harmful relationships, because,

"I probably deserve all this hatred."

The feeling of inadequacy goes beyond even our personal relationships. It spills over into our culture. The sense of inferiority is one reason why money and power have grown to be so important in our society.

When a person is rich and powerful, then there is something tangible to point to as giving worth and esteem. The rich and powerful receive instant admiration just because they are rich and powerful. No other reason but for that. Among other problems, one flaw with that thinking is that there is always at least one other person who has just a little more somewhere in this world. Comparison spells defeat. Acquisitions for the sake of esteem become chains of the prison of inferiority.

"By golly, my kids will have only the best, no matter what it takes. I'm going to provide for my family. They will never have a moment of shame with their clothes, cars, or the house we live in." David promised as he gazed at his firstborn. "They'll never know the embarrassment which I knew growing up on the wrong side of town. I'll be such a good father, they'll never want for anything."

He spent the next eighteen years working at that goal. Designer jeans. His kids had them. Designer tennis shoes. His kids had them. Dance lessons, voice lessons, little league, whatever was in vogue as "THE" activity was what he gave his children. Keeping up with the Joneses was no joke to him. HIS kids not only had to have the best, they had to have it first, before anyone else. When they didn't, he took it personally. He felt that somehow he hadn't been a good enough man, a good enough provider for his family, and had allowed his family to appear inadequate because of his shortcomings. So, he felt hounded to continually make a larger paycheck. That made David feel better about himself. He insisted that his wife work so they could afford the "right" house. His house was the best in town until the doctor decided to custom build himself a new home. Then, David's was no longer the largest and the fanciest. The result was that David's esteem based upon a material possession had lessened.

His children fed the frantic anxiety of the esteem game. Experiencing it themselves, they demanded the same from their father to help chase away the generational shadows of inferiority. It became tragic. The 15 year old daughter wouldn't date anyone who wasn't a letterman and a senior. The older boyfriends had an expensive price tag. They demanded her morals as payment. She turned up pregnant.

The oldest son just couldn't live up to his father's expectations to be perfect. Using the easy-come money from his father, he found acceptance with some druggie friends.

Proverbs 14:12 (NIV) says, **"There is a way that seems right to a man, but in the end it leads to death."**

David's marriage barely survived, but he ended up with a nervous breakdown, no closer to his dream of being the best and having the best for his family. A sad but common story in our nation today.

Advertisers love to leech onto people like this. Using their products as esteem builders, they capitalize on the crippling desire to be good enough. Television pushes this materialistic philosophy. To be worthwhile, buy the best, wear the newest, own the most expensive, and then we might all be worthwhile.

Feelings of inferiority can be seen in other areas as well. It plays a role in the arena of achievement. With an over-achiever the wounded child heart declares, "I'm not good enough so I have to do even more than the average person in order to be worthwhile. I must work harder, give more expensive presents, do more than anyone else just in order to prove my value."

The same problem, but at the other end of the spectrum, is the underachiever. In an underachiever, the wounded child heart says, "I will not put myself in a position of importance because I don't want others to ignore me and make me feel even more insignificant that I already am."

Underachievers are like the man in the parable who hides his talent by burying it. They never live up to their abilities and potential. They waste what God has given them because they walk in fear of success and fear of failure. If this person does try, that fear debilitates to such a degree that failure is inevitable. The lies propagate and feed themselves. Failure is expected, so failure results.

Inferiority breeds inferiority. Children model after their parents' behavior. That's how they learn. That's who they act the most like. If we parents have had trouble with feelings of inferiority then it's time to get rid of them, before our kids absorb any more of the poisonous self-hatred. If our children are displaying a low self-esteem, then we as parents need to look very closely at our own lives. It is very likely that it spilled out of our lives onto our little ones. As parents, we need to daily confess the preciousness and importance of our children in order to begin to break the iron-clad grip of inferiority.

Inferiority is a perversion of godly humility. Humbling ourselves before the Lord results in His lifting us into His arms in a true security. He shows us who we are in Him.

2. HIGH-MINDED INSECURITY

Ever been around someone who has to be right all of the time? He can't stand to be told he might be mistaken or wrong. Some of us have felt this way. It is very difficult to make changes, even in our opinions, because we have to be right in everything. Insecurity demands it. It's very scary to think that we might have made a mistake. We use high-mindedness as a defense mechanism to put a lid on the insecurity in our lives.

Always having to be right in our own eyes is from an ugly, oppressing spirit. It is definitely not from God. In fact, He gives us the truth on this in Prov. 12:15 (NIV) which says, **"The way of a fool seems right to him, but a wise man listens to advice."**

This behavior keeps us from receiving all of the emotional healing we need. There's a fear to admit that we might need some help. Then people would discover we had some inadequacies; that we weren't perfect.

A subtle form of unforgiveness, insecurity grows so strong that forgiving oneself for making even simple mistakes is impossible. There is a great pressure to be right all the time. The unforgiveness grows very dangerous and unpleasant. It's a prison.

High-mindedness is very cruel. If a person is perceived to be of a 'lower class', then the high-minded person allows sarcasm, superiority, and impatience to slip out in their personal dealings. What a perversion! Usually those people who are involved in a life of service are falsely perceived as 'lower class'. God has called all of us to a life of service. How often those who serve, waiters, maids, custodians, teachers, any who are in the helping vocations, are berated with cruel, thoughtless, and unkind attitudes and words! This ugliness feeds the high-mindedness of the one person and the feelings of inferiority in the other. It produces one of those vicious traps satan uses to entangle our lives.

Maybe an astro-physicist justifies high-mindedness because of his mental capacities. It really doesn't matter. Justifiable or not, it is still a sin. It is an attitude which needs repentance because it is placing self above Jesus. Jesus is the only One who is always right. He never makes anyone else feel inferior because of His holiness or goodness. Instead, His attitude of love causes others to be more like Him. That difference right there eliminates the perversion of the defense mechanism of high-mindedness.

3. STUBBORNNESS

Although for a few, stubbornness may be the only defense mechanism in operation in their lives, it is usually tied in with high-minded insecurity. It keeps us from being vulnerable and open to one another as well as being open and vulnerable to the Lord.

Those of us who suffer from this are adamant that everything we do is always right, and everybody else is always wrong. That attitude does not lend itself to trustful interaction among the brethren.

Louis and Carol ministered to one couple who refused to compromise on anything. Each of them was afraid of becoming like the other. Both were critical and judged one another. Stubbornly refusing to entertain anyone else's ideas, they were destroying each other. Stubbornness kept them from receiving healing in their marriage. Nothing was ever achieved.

Ugly stubbornness blocks repentance. It blocks the flow of God as well as blocking people from moving closer to God. It cements the other defense mechanisms to the soul with a super glue. If we have any of the defense mechanisms, but particularly high-minded insecurity, it is entirely possible that stubbornness is hiding in there also.

To set our hearts right before God is the response to stubbornness as the Psalmist says in Chapter 78 Verse 8: (NIV) **"They would not be like their forefathers--a stubborn and rebellious generation, whose hearts were not loyal to God, whose spirits were not faithful to him."**

4. AGGRESSIVE BEHAVIORS.

When we think of aggression, we think of boxing matches, punches thrown, and bodies broken. But, aggressive behaviors include more than the usual expected physical actions. It includes verbal aggression as well. Lashing out, cutting people down, sarcasm, speaking negative words, swearing, put-downs, one-upmanship; all are aggressive behaviors. All wound. All can bring emotional bleeding. All originate from a wounded child heart.

Of course aggression can be physical. Slapping, punching, and hitting out of frustration, come from a feeling of powerlessness, a need for power. Controlling the environment is very important to those who have the defense mechanism of aggression.

It is easy to give vent to anger, indignation and hatred as we go about our daily activities. It is also easy to deeply bury our wrath and hostility and act as if nothing is wrong until in a time of stress it explodes. Neither of these is easy to live with in ourselves or another.

A hostile response to the ups and downs of everyday life opens the door to poor physical health as well as damaging relationships. Because there is often a basic assumption of malice or intentional hurt from other people, it makes it difficult to work out differences and misunderstandings.

Mental health counselors know that when a company closes and there are a lot of lay-offs, that incidents of child abuse skyrocket. The parent strikes out at the child, a weaker person, in frustration at not being able to control his personal environment. Is that reaction, that defense mechanism of aggression, trusting God to take care of every financial situation? Of course not. Those feelings come from a fear-base deep in the wounded child heart. That early pain hinders the growth of trust because of early fears. Those fears in turn foster the growth of defense mechanisms such as aggression.

As mentioned earlier, there are several types of aggression. Bitterness, venom and hatred are forms of emotional aggressiveness, as are pushiness and manipulation. However, they can hide under a passive mask so that everything will appear peaceful.

In the natural, it appears that the active aggressions are far worse than the passive types. We can see the blood. The bruises and broken bones are very visible. But passivity or passive-aggression as it should be called is extremely deceptive. It just appears to be weak. Actually, it's as ugly, vicious, and dangerous as any knock-down drag-out fight. It is deadly. Furthermore, it's killing nature is very easily internalized.

To feel hopeless and helpless is to think that we can't control anything that's going on around us. It draws a pattern of never challenging anything that needs to be dealt with. Walls grow up around everything in this person's life until one slowly withdraws from the process of living. Rage turns inward. A person's soul brutalizes itself.

Passive/aggression developed in Carol's life. She grew very withdrawn from life. She hid behind a shell of romance books. Since she couldn't handle the realities of life she needed a fantasy world where everything was easy and lovely, and had a happily ever-after ending.

After she received healing for her child heart, she had to deal very strongly with passivity. The Lord revealed to her that the "patience" she was so proud of was in many instances passivity. Then, He taught her to recognize the difference between resting in the Lord and aggressive based inactivity.

A victim mentality grows out of the passive/aggression mode. Look at any school playground. It's easy to pick out the child who has begun to live a victim personification. His perception of himself is fulfilled by the ways others pick on him. Watch him walk back into the school building. Never looking at others directly, he averts his eyes and his listless little shoulders slump in anticipation of physical and verbal slurs. Victims see everything and everybody as bigger than they are, and of course much more powerful. It can even develop to where some victims use their victimization to feed their need for power as well as the need to feel special and unique. Being a victim makes them stand out from the crowd.

How many times have we heard someone say, "Well, you know me. It's just my luck that these kind of things happen to me. If I didn't have bad luck, I'd have no luck whatsoever. Poor, poor me. Bad things just follow me around." In the words of Job (6:2,3 NIV) **"If only my anguish could be weighed and all my misery be placed on the scales! It would surely outweigh the sand of the seas."**

They get their attention through the aggression that has been allowed to come against them. Why fix the car when the oil light comes on? Keep on driving it, and it will break down. Then everyone will have to feel sorry and there will be a lot of attention generated. It is manipulation in a hidden, backroads manner.

Victims not only attract problems, they also attract other victims. Then they operate from the shame of whom they are and whom they hang around. Worthlessness and the anticipation of defeat denies the identity for the Believer in Christ Jesus. It denies the power and love of Christ. It also denies the resurrection because in the resurrection there is true power and victory, and an overcoming attitude. Aggression is no longer necessary.

I Cor 13:12 (NIV) assures us, "**Now we see but a poor reflection as in a mirror; then we shall see face to face. Now I know in part; then I shall know fully, even as I am fully known.**" As we seek this face to face, rib to rib relationship with the Holy Spirit, He will teach us day by day who we are and how Jesus sees us!

5. PHYSICAL ILLNESSES

Stress-related illnesses account for the majority of job absenteeism. Having a stress related illness shows what a martyr and hard worker the individual is. For the individual, it proves his worth. After all, he is such a good person, a valuable employee, or a wonderful parent, that he has made himself ill because he works so hard. This induces guilt in others for allowing it to take place and taking advantage of him. It creates a great deal of attention for the sick person. It makes him the center of the universe. Maybe, a family member will give him extra love. When it's a child, perhaps mommy and daddy will spend some time with the little tyke. With adults, chronic illness is a sign that something is spiritually out of whack. They get a temporary sense of acceptance and care that was somehow missed from an earlier time. Used to compensate for the missed-out attention, neglect, and sense of rejection from childhood, illness tries to make up for the pain from the wounding of the little child heart. Although this pattern can continue unto death, it usually does not, because then there would not be any more attention forthcoming for that type of behavior. Hear the age old cry **"My life is consumed by anguish and my years by groaning; my strength fails because of my affliction, and my bones grow weak."** (Psalms 31:10 NIV)

God not only can heal the illness, He can heal the cause of the illness. He can fill the emptiness with His love and His security. Not all illnesses and diseases are caused by a wounded child heart. However, those which are considered stress-related usually are.

6. COMPULSIVE/OBSESSIVE BEHAVIORS

The rejection from childhood still influences the behavior of today. With a wounded child heart, we are under a great deal of stress in our own lives. Self-criticism as well as a critical attitude towards the world sometimes can almost eat us alive. The drive for over-achievement and perfection festers like a blister in our souls. No matter how good a job we do, it feels like we should always do better. For some of us the best is never good enough, which in turn means we are never really good enough. We feel we have to work harder and harder. Then, and only then will we feel worthwhile. It develops into workaholism. Cross addictions come with it.

The obsessive-compulsive, whether it be with alcohol, drugs, food, sex, work, emotions, crises, or gambling might give everything he has to his job. If he is still functioning (not crashed at home, in a treatment center, or just given up on life) he works hard, often coming in early and staying late. Work goes home with him. Work gives him validation, until the obsession overcomes him. Then he's not even a good employee.

Compulsive/obsessive behavior is used to fill an empty hole of desperation which cannot be filled except by a healing from the Lord God Himself. He is the One who brings genuine unconditional love and acceptance as well as value to a person's life.

Anything can become a compulsion. Eating, drinking, drugs, gambling, sex, chronic emotional problems, working, cleaning, shopping, sloppiness, and a drive for perfectionism in self and in others, fall under the compulsive behavior category. Outgrowths of compulsions and obsessions include self-pity, hypersensitivity to the needs of self as well as others, impulsiveness, lack of perseverance, a need for total control and structure, a fear of intimacy, and a need for constant drama and excitement. They dictate a lifestyle that shackles the emotions and limits freedom.

Compulsive behaviors are very serious. They are extremely addictive. Ask any anorexic, alcoholic, or gambler. It is almost an impossibility to stop that behavior in our own strength. Is it difficult for a workaholic executive to go camping with the family without a car phone? Absolutely. Can a junkie pass up a fix? Only with great difficulty. And don't even try to interrupt a bulemic's binge.

Compulsive/obsessive behaviors do not really improve on their own. They are progressive diseases. They get worse as time passes. The addiction deepens. Not only does the body, soul, and spirit of the individual suffer, the entire family structure suffers as he gives his all to his god of compulsion. The entire cycle on some level will probably be repeated into the next generation. This will happen even if no one knows about the compulsiveness; even if the disease has been kept in the "closet", and no one has known about it. It will still show up in subsequent generations. That is because only the symptoms, the compulsiveness, has been hidden. The root cause, the wounded child heart has not been treated.

"For whatever is hidden is meant to be disclosed, and whatever is concealed is meant to be brought out into the open." (Mark 4:22 NIV)

The disease is passed on because the parent is consumed with the obsession rather than with the Lord. The next trip off the wagon is more important than providing a covering of nurture for his children. In order for the obsession to be uprooted and put to rest, the child heart must be made whole.

7. PERFORMANCE

Tying in with compulsive behaviors is perfectionism. Many of us come to believe at a very early age that we must do everything right or perfectly, for if we don't, something terrible will happen. Some of us enter families where tensions are already high and we do not want to add any more stress, less we be the cause of things falling apart.

Others are in situations that are so unstable that we buy the underlying message that somebody (us, of course) has to steady the sinking ship.

The drive to be perfect, to not make any mistakes, or to always be "right" comes from a deeply felt insecurity. Some of the other attitudes already described are responses to this. Perceiving the impossibility of perfection, and feeling overwhelmed by the expectation of it, it is easy to go totally to the other extreme of never trying. The response can be compulsive perfection in some areas and total disarray in other areas of our lives.

Many try so hard to do everything right that when we are confronted with a mistake, we feel our world is shattered. The freedom to say "I was wrong" is one of the greatest freedoms Jesus gives us. He said in Matt. 5:25 (JNT), **"If someone sues you, come to terms with him quickly..."** When anyone says to us "You were wrong" it is so wonderful to be secure enough to respond, "Very likely". We can respond this way because we know that Jesus has paid the price for all our mistakes. He forgives us and enables us to grow and change. We don't have to defend ourselves when we have an advocate who is always defending us with His righteousness. Gal 2:20 (NIV) reads, **"I have been crucified with Christ and I no longer live, but Christ lives in me. The life I live in the body, I live by faith in the Son of God who loved me and gave himself for me."**

8. FEAR

One of the attitudes which causes us much harm is fear and anxiety. God's promise is, **"Whoso harkeneth unto me shall dwell safely, and shall be quiet from fear of evil."** (Prov 1:33 KJV) and **"For God hath not given us a spirit of fear, but of power, and of love, and of a sound mind."** (II Tim. 1:7 KJV) As we come closer to Jesus, He shows us the attitudes of anxiety, nervousness, and worry which are rooted in fear. He also shows us that He is faithful to care for us, that He is always with us and that we can totally trust Him to be there for us. The Lord says in Isa. 57:11 (KJV), **"And of whom hast thou been afraid or feared, that thou hast lied, and hast not remembered me?"** What could happen in our circumstances that are too big for GOD?

Fear will drive us to have some very strange attitudes. We fear intimacy, thinking we will lose our identity, or that if we get too close to someone, they will find out what we are really like. Because of fear we cover up our negative feelings, rather than deal with them. We sometimes believe that if we open up to someone emotionally that they will destroy us. We are afraid of being too close or of being abandoned.

One fear that drives many is fear of losing control of their lives. The Lord indicated to Carol that we haven't any idea what is going on most of the time, much less have the capacity to control events or force things to change. We are far better off to let Him be in charge of our lives.

An attitude is only a way of looking at things. In and of themselves they do not establish facts. Everyone recognizes that a pessimist and an optimist see the same event from opposite perspectives. One sees the glass of water half empty and the other sees it as half full. One viewpoint dictates unhappiness, the other gives a possibility of happiness. We need to check out our attitudes and behaviors to see that they correspond with HIS way of seeing and doing things.

Attitudes are played out in our behaviors. Some, however, are so hidden they are not recognized until we begin to be honest before God and with ourselves.

9. SELF PITY

Another very prevalent attitude in our culture is self-pity. "Oh! poor me" is heard on every side. If we have problems or are distressed, this is an opportunity for our God to show who He is! He gives many instructions to praise in the midst of trouble. Changing how we relate to Him will change the way we look at circumstances. We cannot be in any position now or have been through anything in the past that Jesus considers too much for Him to handle. He has loved us through it all and had His eye on us. (Heb. 13:5 KJV) **"Let your conversation be without covetousness; and be content with such things as ye have: for He hath said, I will never leave thee, nor forsake thee."**

Self-pity manifests itself as it keeps us from recognizing our own accountability for our actions, attitudes or motives. If we excuse ourselves from stewardship, prayer, self-control or forgiveness, we are not responding to the instructions of our Father. "Too tired", "too hurt", "too busy", "too angry", and so on are familiar excuses for not responding to Biblical directions for a godly walk. Then problems pile up until they are overwhelming.

10. PRIDE

One very harmful attitude is that of being better than others. This can range from a secret feeling of superiority to brazen arrogance. All of this is rooted in pride. The Scripture assures us that God **"resisteth the proud and giveth grace to the humble"** (I Pet. 5:5 KJV). Pride erects a facade to show others, that we know enough to control our own lives, to control others, to push and shove our way, to say hurtful and hard things, and to resist new ways of looking at things. This attitude will have us lie to make ourself look "OK" or put others down so that we look better by comparison.

One excellent example is Jesus' familiar story of the Pharisee and the Publican. One was bragging to God about how good he was, how he was so much better than other men! The other was humbling himself before God seeking His mercy, and received peace. It concludes with this, **"For everyone who exalts himself will be humbled, and he who humbles himself will be exalted."** (Luke 18:14 NIV)

We all come to a place where God will begin to deal with us in this area. Do we resist the Word? We assure ourselves that we "know better" or want to "decide for ourselves". Pride can even lead us to decide that God doesn't mean what He says!

The Word of God says in Proverbs that pride goes before a fall. James 4:6 (NIV), also states,

"God opposes the proud
but gives grace to the humble."

God is gracious to warn us of the serious consequences of lifting ourselves up in our own estimation. After all wasn't this what Lucifer did? We can ask the Lord to show us our own heart attitudes in this area so that we need not crash in defeat.

11. GREED/LUST

Some of us find ourselves trying to fill up the emptiness of our lives with all kinds of things. A consuming overwhelming drive, greed and lust cause us to behave in a way that is wrong in order to obtain what appears to be fulfilling. We will even do things that we know deep in our heart are very wrong. However, the fulfillment we seek is always elusive. We desire more...and more...and more.

"From the least to the greatest,
all are greedy for gain;
prophets and priests alike,
all practice deceit.
They dress the wound of my people
as though it were not serious.
'Peace, peace' they say,
when there is no peace." (Jer. 6:13,14 NIV)

Neither the grasping of material goods nor carnal pleasures can ever satisfy the deep needs we have. God gives us legitimate needs and He alone knows how to fill them. Trying to supply them ourselves from an illegitimate source (one other than God) only brings more emptiness.

The Word of God can transform our old thought patterns so that we can begin to trust His faithfulness. Our hearts need to be turned toward God as our "needs meeter". The foundation of the Word can be stolen from us if we do not allow it to have leverage in our lives. **"Still others, like seed sown among thorns, hear the word; but the worries of this life, the deceitfulness of wealth and the desires for other things come in and choke the word, making it unfruitful."** (Mark 4:18,19 NIV)

12. IMPATIENCE/HURRY

Getting the cart before the horse, we try to live our lives in the fast lane. We fail to put priorities in the best order and try to construct a life structure without an adequate foundation. We fail to deal with one problem before we plunge into another. All of us know people who cannot seem to complete any chore, and whose daily activities pile up until they appear impossible.

Most of us are in a big hurry to get what we want -- instead of wanting to wait for God's plan for our lives to blossom. We attempt to rush faster and faster to do more and more only to accomplish less and less. Then we are frustrated to a point of franticness.

In Scripture, peace and patience are both given as fruit of the Spirit (Gal 5:22 above). It is **"through faith and patience [that we] inherit what has been promised"** (Heb. 6:12 NIV). If our daily lives are 'out of sync' with the peace of God, we can, through His grace, begin to experience it.

13. LASCIVIOUSNESS

"Lasciviousness" is a word that the Lord spoke to Louis a few weeks after He began to show Louis what was resident in Louis' heart. It meant that he was self-indulgent and did not control his eating as well as other habits. There was a high price to pay for not dealing with this behavior.

When Jesus went to the cross, the Scripture says that He bought us. When we accept Him as Savior, we begin to walk in a different covenant than the world and are accountable to Him for our obedience to His Word. Taking care of our bodies and being temperate in our habits are instructions found in many places in the Word. **"Don't you know that you yourselves are God's temple and that God's Spirit lives in you? If anyone destroys God's temple, God will destroy him; for God's temple is sacred, and you are that temple."** (I Cor. 3:16-17 NIV) God cared enough for the children of Israel that He gave them dietary instructions. He provided food, water, clothing, and heating and air-conditioning during their forty year trek through the desert. He cares that much and more for us. **"For God so loved the world, that he gave his only begotten Son, that whosoever**

believeth in him should not perish, but have everlasting life" (John 3:16 KJV).

So much burden lifts from us when we begin to let Jesus be the Lord of what we eat, what we say, how we drive, when we do things, and so on. Frustration fades and then vanishes when He is consulted about details of our life. We can be satisfied with an alternate standard of living when He brings peace to our hearts. Instead of filling the wounded child heart with indulgences, we can let the Lord fill the ache, and it will be healed.

When we are born again the Lord comes to live inside us. Phil. 4:13 (KJV) reminds us, **"I can do all things through Christ which strengthens me".** The Lord will work in us to guide and direct us to better choices.

14. ENVY

One of the most deceptive attitudes we can allow to grow is one of envy, jealousy, or covetousness. We are always looking across the fence at someone else's "greener pasture". The Lord recognized this inclination in our fleshly nature and considered it serious enough to address in the 10th Commandment. Ex. 20:17 (NIV) reads, **"You shall not covet your neighbor's house. You shall not covet your neighbor's wife, or his manservant or maidservant, his ox or donkey, or anything that belongs to your neighbor."**

The practice of always wishing our circumstances or our physical makeup were different is a very typical mind set of many people. The Lord desires that we look to Him and Him only as our source, and to trust His wisdom for our lives. We can choose to accept our circumstances as an opportunity to grow in our trust in God, or we can flail about in rebellion or resentment.

Many people resent their own appearance. "I wish my nose looked like Jane's!" "Why can't I be taller?" Beginning in childhood we check how we look in every mirror or plate glass window we pass by. We gripe and complain about the "faults" we see there. The Lord likes our unique individuality. We are all beautiful to Him! When we can accept ourselves we will also be healthier! The Scriptures indicate that our heart attitudes affect our health. One specific area is that **"envy rots the bones"** as we are informed in Prov. 14:30 (NIV).

Our Father has good plans for us. We need to put our hand in His, and let Him lead us. When we are jealous of another we are questioning God's wisdom. Do our brothers or sisters seem to have a favored place? Does one spouse have it easier than the other? Do friends have less responsibility at their jobs than we do, yet earn more? Do the things which are difficult for us seem to be so easy for our neighbors? Release these things to the Lord. Set our eyes upon Him! He is the source of all favor. Psalm 73 is an excellent promise that regardless of what is going on in others' lives, we can turn to God for His special provision suited to us. Prov. 3:5,6 (NIV) instructs, **"Trust in the Lord with all your heart and lean not on your own understanding; in all your ways acknowledge him and he will make your paths straight".**

15. APATHY

The picture of the believer painted in the New Testament is of an on-fire, active follower of the Master. This portrays one whose life is radically changed by meeting Jesus. Apathy about our relationship with the Lord or laziness in being about the Father's business does not fit this criteria. Being undependable in our daily lives, and passive about changing life patterns results from being deeply wounded.

There is no place for slothfulness in a believer indwelt by the Spirit of the living God! Prov. 6:9-10 (NIV) points out, **"How long will you lie there, you sluggard? When will you get up from your sleep? A little sleep, a little slumber, a little folding of the hands to rest -- and poverty will come on you like a bandit and scarcity like an armed man."**

The Christian life is one of action. The main thrust of our activity is going toward Jesus, being directed by the Holy Spirit. Secondarily, we withstand the forces of darkness. If inaction is a problem in our lives it is likely that healing is needed to lift the heaviness which weighs us down. As healing begins to take place we will find ourselves able to enter into worship and warfare. Entering the Christian life is akin to joining the "green berets" corps. Healing precedes the ability to take back territory from the enemy, so healing must take place.

Procrastination also falls under the heading of apathy. We live today! The Bible says, **"now is the day of salvation"** (II Cor. 6:2 KJV), and **"in the day of salvation I**

will help you". (Isa. 49:8 NIV) The Lord must be allowed to guide us and direct us today in what we are to accomplish.

16. DENIAL

Denying problems and denying reality, is a way of coping for many wounded people. It is a way of life. If we have only a dysfunctional family as our standard, we have no foundation from which to build. Once we begin to stand on the Rock, we can begin to deal with problems. We have a safe place to retreat as things which have terrified us in the past are once more attacking us. We do not have to rely on our own strength. We can safely look at things differently.

Some of us are just too stubborn to admit we have had a faulty view of life. Others of us have trained our souls not to register hurts consciously or not to "see" what is going on in our lives.

Louis and Carol were so involved in a religious system which taught denial that it took some intensive retraining by the Word to walk free of it. They had accepted a teaching for years which denied that God acknowledged their natural lives. This teaching played havoc in their marriage relationship. It was a wonderful deliverance to find that the Lord was very interested in every detail of our lives.

17. NEGATIVITY

One of the favorite ploys of the enemy of our souls is to train us to be negative. We will learn to criticize, to expect the worst, to downgrade good things, to plan to fail. We feel we are not worthwhile enough to have blessings from God in our lives. We are even suspicious if things are going well, the bottom is about to fall out of our lives. Nothing is quite good enough -- either ourselves, or our circumstances, or our blessings.

This mind set is diametrically opposed to walking in the joy of the Lord. It is the opposite of faith and trust in His goodness. As we turn toward the Lord and begin to speak with our mouths and believe in our hearts that He is a faithful, loving God who cares for us, our heart attitudes begin to change toward new directions.

We need healing in our child heart. For this to happen, we need to recognize our symptoms which are fed by that pain. Although several major behavioral and attitude problems have been discussed, they are not the only ones. Others include an unnatural super-concern of the welfare of animals. (The person relates to the helplessness of small animals as well as a fear of intimacy with people.) Excessive talking is a problem which hides the fear that the individual might hear something negative as well as keeping painful memories at bay. And the list goes on. We need to seek our hearts honestly for anything that is a result of deep rejection, anything that is not of God.

When we are wounded we make decisions about ourselves and others and form opinions and have mindsets which are not founded on truth. Jesus said, **"I am the way, the truth and the life: no man cometh unto the Father, but by me."** (John 14:6 KJV) If JESUS is TRUTH, or dependable reality, (and He is!), this certainly needs to affect our viewpoint!

God wants to set us free of all of those defense mechanisms so that we can be single-minded and serve the Lord Jesus Christ. He wants us at peace, no longer struggling with the storms of our emotions or the dictates of our defense mechanisms. He wants us healed.

"Then they cried to the Lord in their trouble, and he saved them from their distress. He sent forth his word and healed them; he rescued them from the grave. Let them give thanks to the Lord for his unfailing love and his wonderful deeds for men." (Psalms 107:19-21 NIV)

HEALING

CHAPTER 5

A giant step in the healing process comes with trust. At some point, if we are to get well, we must decide to trust God. Although we may not as yet be convinced we can trust Him, we do come to a time when there is no place else to go. Some of us only reach this point when we have tried every other possible way. It can be a rough road. Jesus reaches out His hand whenever we are ready to accept it.

When we make the decision to accept Him as our answer, progress is continuous. Our healing and freedom is even more important to Him than to us! Redemption -- paying the full price to buy back that which has been lost -- is why He came.

Jesus Christ paid the price for all of us to be free of the terrible hurts caused by a wounded child heart. He paid the price for us to rise with Him through the cross.

II Cor. 8:9 says, "**For you know the grace of our Lord Jesus Christ, that though He was rich, yet for your sakes He became poor, so that you through His poverty might become rich.**" (NIV)

He has paid the price for us to be free of hurts, pains, wrongs, and sins. For every single one of our wounds, He was wounded. He rose again so that as we accept Him, we too can rise with Him. With Jesus we can have a healthy and whole mind, will, and emotions; all of those things that make up the soul.

First, let's clarify what is meant in discussing the heart, spirit, and soul. Heart Menders perceives the "heart" as the "container" for both the spirit -- that part of a reborn person which is in touch with and united with God -- and the soul. The soul is best defined as the mind, will, and emotions. The physical body makes up the third part of man's triune being. They are distinct but united. It is when these parts are at war that there are problems.

Before we commit our lives to God and ask Him to rule our hearts, the soul rules. Our mind, will, and emotions are very well trained in selfishness. Now, they must be retrained to bow their knee to a new Lord!

Our body is greatly influenced positively or negatively by the choices we make in our heart. The Bible teaches that a healthy, peaceful heart -- where the soul is not rebellious -- gives health to our bodies. Prov. 4:20-22 (NIV) says "**My son, pay attention to what I say; listen closely to my words. Do not let them out of your sight, keep them within your heart; for they are life to those who find them**

and health to a man's whole body." The body is to be God's "temple", not at odds with our spirit-ruled life.

As we recognize the difference between the spirit and soul, we can begin to train the soul to cooperate with the guidance of the Holy Spirit.

As most of us have discovered in our lives, the soul and flesh literally war with the spirit man to keep us bound. They definitely do not want to let us walk in freedom. It is only by the Spirit of the Living God that they can even be overcome. It is impossible to accomplish this in the flesh, although many try. That's where a mountain of pride puffs up with "I am tough enough to beat this." "I have enough will power." "I can be good enough."

Self-control alone just doesn't cut it.

Millions of dollars are spent each year in the diet industry for this very reason. Miracle Foods. Behavior Modification. Diet Clubs. Spas. They don't keep people thin. They don't make them happy. The root of the problem, the wounded child heart, is not fixed. Only the symptoms have been addressed. Sure, there are a small number of people who seem to beat their problems. Either they have wrapped their lives around maintaining normality or they have received some type of healing. The twelve step programs have offered healing for thousands who are chained to addictions. Many have been helped, although some others have come under condemnation for even attending the meetings. Others, in the necessary process of accepting responsibility for their own actions, have not gone on to release the sin and accept forgiveness and healing.

We all tend to judge ourselves on the basis that we can handle our own problems.

"If I was just strong enough." "If I just exercised will power." "I could get better, if I would try harder." It's just not true. With only the power of ourselves and others' mental abilities we can't get well. We cannot heal ourselves. We aren't strong enough to conquer our souls, using the soul as the healer, no matter how hard we try.

"For God gave us a Spirit who produces not timidity, but power, love, and self-discipline." (II Timothy 1:7 JNT)

Healing IS possible to people with wounded child hearts. Most of us need some level of healing as we learn to be single minded to serve Jesus. IF we recognize a wounded child heart AND are willing to do what it takes to get to the point of healing, we CAN be healed.

This sounds like an immense project -- to "redo" our entire life! The marvelous part is we have a Helper -- One who has come alongside to be there to teach, to provide answers, to comfort and encourage. When we accept Jesus as our Savior, He sends the Holy Spirit to minister His grace in our lives. Luke 4:18 (KJV) says that Jesus was anointed **"to preach the gospel to the poor; he hath sent me to heal the broken-hearted, to preach deliverance to the captives, and recovery of sight to the blind, to set at liberty them that are bruised"**. Sounds like He had our healing in mind, doesn't it?

When we are born again, the Holy Spirit -- the Spirit of God -- dwells with us and we can be in contact with Him continually. Part of His assignment is found in Jude 24 (NIV); **"To him who is able to keep you from falling and to**

present you before his glorious presence without fault and with great joy". His work is to day by day transform us into the character and likeness of Jesus! We only need to yield to this and cooperate with Him!

One result of this is a continual cleansing process. The word *catharsis* can be defined as *'a purging, cleaning out; to cleanse of moral defilement; freeing the mind from agitation by eliminating all base ideas; healing process by which the mind is cleansed of factors that tend to disrupt mental activities and cause anxiety, anguish or unhappiness. Most of these factors are subconscious thereby including early experiences.'*

The Holy Spirit functions like a master housekeeper. He wants to clean out cupboards and closets and get the dirt and accumulated grime out of corners. He will always ask permission before disposing of "our stuff". Remember, when He shows us another "collection" of "old garbage", that He recognizes garbage when He sees it and knows what it will do to us if we choose to keep it! But He always asks us to choose! He works quietly, gently, but persistently. He never embarrasses us or hurts us. And He is a heart changer. One day the Lord said to Carol, "Until the heart is changed, evil merely changes masks."

To receive healing of the wounded child heart, the Holy Spirit will lead us through processes. Without going through each one of these, the process of healing will be frustrated and will never really be complete. These are essential ways we need to allow the work of the Spirit to retrain our old "soulish" ways of reacting.

THE FORGIVENESS & REPENTANCE PROCESS

1. FORGIVENESS

Most of us are quick to walk away from obvious sins of the flesh. It is the sinful responses in the heart to horrible things which were done to us that are the ones which are hidden, deceptive, and difficult to deal with. It's as if we want to bury these things. They are not to be discussed even if they are known. Usually they are not even recognized. They are suppressed and denied. They aren't dealt with. And if not dealt with, these old life patterns influence every thing we do. They fester in our hearts.

This was the first basic lesson which Louis and Carol had to learn in their own lives. There has to be forgiveness towards those who have hurt us, as well as, and very importantly, towards ourselves. It is critical to forgive in both directions when dealing with the healing of the defensive, wounded child heart.

"Dana", a lovely woman in her early twenties, was shaking as she sat across the desk from Kathryn.

"I just don't know what's wrong with me. I'm not having any success in my life. Well, no that's not true. Things start working out for me, and I just mess them up. I seem headed for failure no matter what I try." She began sobbing.

Dana had been raped several years earlier. Kathryn knew that Dana had forgiven the man who had committed the crime against her. She had already come a long way in her healing. Now, she seemed to be at a standstill in her recovery. It was time to take care of the unfinished business of the rape. Dana was ready to take her healing to the next step. Kathryn discussed the necessity for Dana to forgive herself for being a part of the rape. Even though Dana was the victim, and was not at fault, she still needed to forgive herself for it having happened.

Later, Dana related, "I thought I had taken care of everything when I had forgiven the guy who had done that to me. It never crossed my mind to forgive myself, because I hadn't done anything wrong. But, it makes sense to forgive myself, because I had always carried this load of guilt around. Thoughts like, 'maybe if I had fought harder, or had carried a gun, or hadn't been at that location, this wouldn't have happened to me.' I don't think any of that would have made a difference to what happened, but those thoughts still affected me."

"I needed to forgive myself, innocent as I was. I had to, in order to find the peace that I've been desperately needing. Now, I have the freedom to be successful. I can finally get on with my life. I now see a future for myself. Praise God." She smiles, "I'm at peace with myself. It's wonderful."

Forgiving oneself is very, very hard for most of us. If we were the ones who committed a sin against someone else, it is essential that we receive the forgiveness the Lord provides for us, whatever the sin. Maybe we just did something stupid. Maybe we omitted doing something. Forgiveness is still important for our lives. Accepting forgiveness for ourselves must always take place for healing. We still need to forgive ourselves. When we don't forgive ourselves, we are actually hanging Jesus back up on the tree. We are crucifying Him all over again, because we are denying His Blood the ability to cover our sins, even those sins against ourselves. The first half of the forgiveness process must be the forgiveness of self.

The second part of forgiveness is the forgiving of others. This certainly isn't easy either. Especially when the other person has been so clearly and vilely wrong. However, it MUST be done. The peace of God will always be an elusive dream unless we can walk in forgiveness toward those around us.

To truly forgive by the power in the Name of Jesus is a spiritual transaction which is recorded in heaven. It is more than a mental agreement. It brings eternal and temporal results. It changes dynamics in our relationships toward God and toward people. Further, it requires a follow-through chain of choices in our day to day life from then on. We can begin to live according to the ways of God's love.

A lot of us say, "Okay, Jesus, You can have this area of my life and this area, and oh, all right, you can even have this area over here in this part of my heart, but please keep your hands off my wounded child heart, especially that corner where I'm storing all the offenses that people have committed against me. I mean after all, Jesus, THEY sinned against ME! I'm justified in my anger. I didn't do anything to deserve the way they've treated me. I've been hurt badly, and I still hurt after all this time. Those who have hurt me deserve for me to be angry at them.

"Yes, Jesus, you can be Lord. In fact, I want you to be Lord. But, don't touch my right to get mad at my spouse, or parents, my neighbor, or my children, or

my right to be offended,
my right to pout,
my right to act selfishly,
my right to feel sorry for myself,
my right to explode in anger,
my right to rant and rave, and fly off the handle!"

If Jesus is going to be Lord, <u>and it IS an on-going process,</u> then there are no rights to be clutched onto. Those rights and the whole selfish lifestyle with it should be laid down at the Cross of Calvary. Our old sin nature was nailed to the cross so that we could rise above that as a joint-heir of Christ. Now we get to walk that out daily.

All of us have been bought and purchased by Jesus' blood. None of us have any rights to live that old selfish, soulish lifestyle. This would seem unfair except for the fact that Jesus has paid a high price for our freedom. As we receive HIS ability to restore and heal, we can freely make the appropriate transactions in the Spirit. As we choose to forgive and repent of the judgement we are released from the hurt.

Our response to this is either going to be AMEN or OH ME! The only right we have is to be like Jesus. Before we get uptight, we need to remember we're still way ahead of the unbelievers. Their only right is to be like satan, and quite frankly that is not a privilege at all. Rather it is an enslavement.

A big part of that unforgiveness towards others must include:

1. Parents
2. People in authority

Even children make sinful responses. As we become accountable, we must repent of those childish sinful responses even if they were seemingly made innocently when we were young.

To illustrate forgiving freely, in Matthew 18 Jesus tells a story of a man who was forgiven a vast sum of money by his king and immediately refused to forgive a fellow worker who owed him one day's wages. The king's anger at his refusal to bless as he had been blessed ends with **"And his lord was wroth, and delivered him to the tormentors, till he should pay all that was due unto him. So likewise shall my heavenly Father do also unto you, if ye from your hearts forgive not everyone his brother their trespasses."** (Matt. 18: 34,35 KJV)

When we refuse to learn how to forgive, we will be turned over to the "tormentors." If we are experiencing a great deal of torment, we need look no further. We are probably harboring some kind of unforgiveness in our lives.

"Lee's" heart had been giving him trouble. He had trouble catching his breath, and he just could not get a good night's sleep. He had decided it was time to visit the doctor. He was getting very worried about it.

The week before he planned to go for his check-up, he met with Louis and Carol for some personal ministry. During that process, he forgave many people who had hurt him; people whom he had not thought about for a long, long time. He also forgave his wife who had recently left him. He forgave himself as well.

That night, he slept like a baby. His irregular heart rhythms stopped. He could breathe. He was well. He had forgiven.

Woundedness creates an expectancy of more hurt. Bitter roots grab at the heart and cripple the life. Hebrews 12:15 (NIV) warns, **"See to it that no one misses the grace of God and that no bitter root grows up to cause trouble and defile many."**

Unforgiveness and bitterness can be sins unto death. Following us all the way unto the grave they often take us there early. They bring about physical reactions, which lead to all kinds of infirmities.

Forgiveness is the first step for healing. It includes oneself and others.

2. REPENTANCE

The Hebrew word translated repent is 'nacham'. It pictures a "release of breath" or a letting go. As we "let go" of our self-righteousness we will be free of the old hurts. Interestingly, in the King James Version of the Old Testament, nacham is translated 38 times "repent" and 41 times "comfort". So the release that comes through repentance brings the comfort of the Holy Spirit.

This is the beginning of healing, when we repent and ask His help in overcoming them. Repentance is a big part of God's program. Rom. 2:4 (NIV) says, **"do you show contempt for the riches of his kindness, tolerance and patience, not realizing that God's kindness leads you toward repentance?"**

Repentance softens us toward God so that we are open to His correction. **"...easy to be entreated..."** (James 3:17 KJV)

Repentance prepares our hearts to enter a more productive relationship with the Lord. John the Baptist was sent to prepare the way for the first coming of the Messiah by calling out for repentance. The way is being prepared for His second coming by the purification of the waiting bride. The church is being brought to a place of repentance one way or another.

Most of us have many sins of the heart to repent for. The Holy Spirit is faithful to bring them up for review as we are ready to deal with them. Some of these are unforgiveness which we have called by other names. Being bitter, critical, and easily offended are close kin to unforgiveness. As we see these in our attitudes we will want to tell our Father that we see these sins for what they are and ask His help in cleansing them from our heart.

Jealousy and envy are also heart sins which will need to be repented of.

As we see how the Lord meets us and heals us in repentance, we can begin to recognize the deceptions the enemy has pulled on us!

We will see patterns of denial or fears which had plagued us. When we trust the work of the Holy Spirit in our hearts we will know that as He uncovers a sin He will also minister to us in grace and mercy as we repent. Then the truth of God's Word will replace with hope the areas we thought were beyond an answer.

Quite often we are blind to these heart sins until we commit to repent of what ever God shows us. The tender willingness to repent really opens the door to great amounts of healing. The hardness of self-righteousness prevents our receiving all the healing we need!

As mentioned earlier, those with wounded child hearts need to release from judgement those in authority positions. After that, comes the repentance for sinning against authority. Everyone should take care of this, but those who never seem to get along with bosses need to pay particular attention. If we are one of those who are always bucking the system we need to repent for sinning against authority for attitudes and actions. It takes a transformation of our heart to walk in a godly humility toward those in authority over us.

The healing of the child heart begins with forgiveness and repentance. The necessity of repentance can be seen in the analogy of a cowboy roping a calf.

The calf is like the person who has hurt us. The rope is the unforgiveness that we have towards that person. As long as the cowboy holds onto the rope, he is connected to the calf. We hold on to unforgiveness the same way. The result is that there is always a tie or a bond haunting and bothering both people. It takes releasing the rope through repentance for both to be free. As long as we hang onto that unforgiveness, we will never be free. We will always be burdened by that extra baggage. Our activities and thoughts will be overshadowed by the unforgiveness we insist upon holding. Obviously the rope must be released. **"If you forgive anyone his sins, they are forgiven; if you do not forgive them, they are not forgiven."** (John 20:23 NIV)

Freedom can be achieved by forgiving the person who wronged us, and then repenting for judging them. It's the ol' one, two in heart mending. Repentance is equally important as the act of forgiving. When someone hurts us we usually end up judging them for it. Our judging another person will end up causing us the same problems. **"Do not judge, and you will not be judged. Do not condemn and you will not be condemned. Forgive, and you will be forgiven. Give, and it will be given to you. A good measure, pressed down, shaken together and running over, will be poured into your lap. For with the measure you use, it will be measured to you."** (Luke 6:37-38 NIV) It is not our job to judge those around us. It is our job to walk in love and forgiveness and to trust God.

Repentance is recognizing sin as sin, realizing that we cannot be "good enough" to atone for it, and releasing it to God. God has provided our freedom by the shed Blood of our Lord, Jesus Christ. We can only humble ourselves to receive what He has done for us that we could not do ourselves. The more we see of God's love and His holiness, the less we will defend our mistakes. Prov. 12:15 (KJV) tells us that **"a fool is right in his own eyes".** Until we will humble ourselves and not push our own ways and attitudes, we cannot benefit from the joy of repentance.

Once we understand the importance of forgiveness AND repentance we can begin to receive the healing for our little child hearts. It's now time to go forward from the past. It's time to practice forgiveness and repentance in earnest so that we can be blanketed with healing.

Since so many hurts occur during childhood, it's very likely that there are scores of people we need to forgive and repent of judging. We need to take care of that to experience a whole, completed heart.

Take a couple of quiet hours, and sit down with Jesus. Make sure to be uninterrupted. Then, ask Him to bring all the names and faces of the people we need to forgive for hurting and offending us during the last year until the present time. Just be quiet. The Lord will bring the names, faces, and memories to us. As He does, respond in the following manner. Let's say it was Aunt Mary who really hurt our feelings last week. We would pray, "I forgive Aunt Mary for criticizing me, and I repent of judging her. I ask You to bless Aunt Mary and heal her as well."

We forgive the offender for hurting us. Then we repent of judging the person. Finally, we ask for the peace of God to fill the place where the pain had lived. Speak it aloud. Let our own ears hear the words of forgiveness and repentance that are spoken aloud.

Once that year is cleaned up, go back to the year before that, and cleanse it through forgiveness and repentance.

Clean up several years of life in this way. Then, go back five years at a time until we get to the times when we were born. Ask the Lord to bring the names, faces, and circumstances when we had been hurt. It is truly amazing at how many there are: old playmates, coaches, relatives, former teachers, old boyfriends, old girlfriends, it will probably be quite a list. Particularly investigate the area of close family relationships. Forgive and repent. Don't pick the burdens back up.

This process took Kathryn about a week. She so desired to be wholly healed, that she would wake herself up in the middle of the night, talking out loud, forgiving people in her sleep whom the Father had brought to her sleeping consciousness. But, by the end of the week she was refreshed, whole, and at peace.

First, forgive. Secondly, repent.

3. BECOME CHILDLIKE

"Be imitators of God, therefore, as dearly loved children." (Eph. 5:1 NIV)

While Carol was having quiet time with the Lord, He showed that giving was His activity or expression of Love. That is the exact opposite of what most think. For the majority of us, the view has been that God is wanting to take away and keep things from us. Actually, that reflects how we've grown up feeling about other people.

But, the Lord wants to GIVE. Our needs are channels for His love. The needs in our lives are the points of contact. Faith is believing that God will, is able, and wants to meet our needs, and it becomes the point of contact or point of readiness to receive from Him.

Carol was hung up on whether her needs were legitimate.

"For many years I was my own sufficiency. I met my own needs and took care of myself, all the while pushing down feelings of overwhelming inadequacy. The devil could always convince me that if it was my need then it probably was not a real 'need'. I was really worked over by the enemy."

The question is not if a need is legitimate or not. If it is a perceived need on our part, then God wants to deal with it on our behalf.

Hebrews 11:6 (KJV) says, **"Without faith it is impossible to please him; for he that cometh to God must believe that he is and that he is a rewarder of them that diligently seek him."**

As we seek Him, He will give us the reward of meeting our needs. By pouring Himself out, God is giving to His people.

Carol continues, "If I had no needs, then I would have no need of God. To think that I had no need of anything is totally selfish. Although I had tried to be totally sufficient without leaning on God, I never realized how I needed Him. It just did not work. I could never relax. I never felt really calm and peaceful. The facade of having it all together was a shaky lie. Everything was always at the brink of crashing down about my ears. The Lord wants me to need Him. In fact, He needs me to need Him. I'm reminded of an illustration that Malcolm Smith relates: that we should think of ourselves as baby birds with mouths open waiting to be fed by a generous, giving God who desires to fill our hunger."

To be like a child who is walking, even running, but all the while holding onto the Father's hand, fully trusting the Father to keep him safe, is the way we need to see ourselves. Checking to see if something is okay to do, asking permission easily with no self-will, and trusting His "say-so" all show a whole heart directed towards the Lord. He doesn't want us childish, but truly childlike.

To be **"poor in Spirit"** (Matt. 5:3) means to realize that we are nothing without the Lord. We can expect God to meet us at our point of need because it is His nature to do so. If we were to be sufficient without Him, we would have no needs. The recognition of the totality of our needs is part of the laying down of self.

This revelation was a major step in the transformation of Carol's life. She is now much more able to believe Him to meet her needs.

The uniqueness of God is His ability to meet every person's needs all the time. He is so able and eager to pour out His love for everyone, that He gives us the ability to repent and ask for forgiveness. When we come to Him at our points of need, He forgives us. He accepts us.

4. REDEFINING OURSELVES THROUGH THE WORD

A baby develops the image of himself from others. It comes from what parents think about him. Whether the words spoken to him are put-downs or statements of acceptance and admiration, they build the child's picture of himself. He looks in a mirror through other people's eyes.

We rebuild and grow our child heart by looking in the mirror of the Word of God. When we look in the Word, we see how Jesus sees us. This is how we are to see ourselves as well. Reassuring ourselves of who we are with these promises of God, we can spot the devices of the enemy as they come against us. We've heard some of them many times during our lives.

"You can't be successful. You can't achieve that. You'll never be anything. You're no good."

When we know the Word, all of that garbage can be challenged. Remind satan as well as ourselves, "God says that I'm **'accepted in the beloved'**" (Eph. 1:6) that Jesus will never leave me or forsake me. (Heb. 13:5)

We can nourish our child heart as we would feed an infant. Feed it the life giving milk of the Scriptures. Feed it the meat of the Word. Jesus wants us to see ourselves as He does.

What God's Word says is from the Tree of Life. What our five natural senses tell us is from the Tree of the Knowledge of Good and Evil.

When "Jo's" husband ran off and left her, her mind centered on her circumstances. She felt that she had a right to be angry. She was hostile as well as very hurt.

When Sunday came around, she went to church and heard the Word of God. It sharply contrasted with the hard feelings that she had been fighting all week. She experienced a short, vicious battle within herself. Even before she made it to the church parking lot, all of the hurt, betrayal, and anger pushed back up to the forefront.

Clearly Jo had a divided heart. When we allow our soul (the mind, will, and emotions) to govern us because we are focusing on the circumstances, we won't have any heart peace. It is not possible. We are looking through worldly glasses. Jo discovered that focusing on the circumstances made her feel like her guts were being ripped apart because they conflicted with the Word. Focusing on the circumstances will tear us up every time. We must focus on what the Word says, NOT the circumstances!

"For let not that man think that he shall receive anything of the Lord. A double-minded man is unstable in all his ways. (James 1:7,8 KJV)

The reverse is also true. A single minded man can expect everything. That is one very good reason why the child heart must get healed. We all must become single-minded about what God's Word says.

When wounded reasoning and the unrenewed mind look only at circumstances, they will argue with the Word of God. We must tell ourselves, "No! Shut down soul. You must cooperate with my spirit man. I'm going straight to God's Word to find out what I can trust."

This is NOT denial of reality. Reality IS the Word of God. Our opinions fluctuate. Circumstances are constantly altering. God is unchanging. God is God!

The eye cannot be single if we look at the circumstances. Seeing how rotten the situation is and mulling it over in our mind is so easy. On the other hand, to seek out God's Word to see what it has to say about it requires discipline. Why does trying to learn the Lord's viewpoint and walk in His Word pull so hard against the information from reasoning and circumstances?

For all these years we've trusted in our perceptions; that little computer bank of knowledge, both of good and evil, that has been fed into our minds since day one. Covering what looks good, what looks bad, what tastes good, what tastes bad, what we think will work and what won't work, we're trained to look at everything by our limited reasoning.

Matthew 6:24 (KJV) says, "**No man can serve two masters: for either he will hate the one and love the other; or else he will hold to the one and despise the other. Ye cannot serve God and mammon.**"

Mammon is what we trust in, what we live for, what we wrap our lives around -- what we worship. The hurts and offenses in our lives easily become "mammon" when the child heart is wounded. This is IDOLATRY! Forgiveness and repentance puts the idol where it belongs -- under our feet!

Vacillating between the Lord and circumstances, the child heart will stay torn. We need to be single-minded. Our eyes must stay on the Lord.

This requires discipline. It requires a disciplining to choose Jesus. According to Vine's Concordance, 'discipline' is 'the saving of the mind'. The mind is part of the soul along with the will and emotions.

An example would be "Mary Jo" who was raised in a dysfunctional family. Her bitterness caused her to build walls of resentment. She continued to hold on to the old images of her family members, even after others in the family had been drawn to the Lord and had experienced repentance and great healing, and now loved Mary Jo unconditionally. As she came to the Lord, she had to make a choice. Because of her new love for Jesus, she had to choose to see her family members as He did. Then she, too, was able to receive healing.

Lay aside the old man, put on the new.

Start thinking in new Jesus ways. Agree that the Word is Truth.

Start acting in new life-giving ways. Act on what the Word says.

Look at old thoughts and patterns and measure them by the Word. In the Word, God shows us what His patterns are for our lives.

One of the ways we have found to break through the bondage of shame and guilt is to take the person in front of a mirror. As they look themselves in the eye, we lead them through speaking out a recognition of who they are in Christ Jesus. According to the Word of God, forgiveness and repentance is part of this redefining.

As we get ready for our healing, we might wonder just what normal behavior is. Some of us have never been exposed to normal, healthy behavior. We must look to Jesus. He gives us a wonderful example of normality. Jesus doesn't expect us to be perfect. He took care of that by being perfection. He did His human time on this planet in a perfect manner and He just expects us to allow Him to live through us. But, it's not by our performance or in our own strength that we are to live. It is through Him and His strength which allows us to achieve higher ground in the Spirit. **"I was crucified with Christ, nevertheless I live; yet not I, but Christ liveth in me: and the life that I now live in the flesh I live by the faith of the Son of God who loved me, and gave himself for me."** (Gal. 2:20 KJV)

The Lord who brings us liberty will set us free as we begin to get the image of ourselves from the mirror of the Spirit of God. By searching the Scriptures to see who we are in Christ Jesus, we will begin to be conformed to this new image. There is no room in this new image for old thinking. It does not include being wounded, being a chronic victim, or having a lifetime of garbage still attached. Jesus has come to set us free from all of that. And He will!

Healing requires forgiveness and repentance. It requires becoming childlike and redefining ourselves in the Word. It requires a willingness to let go of the "self" we've always been familiar with.

This release will bring a triumph of healing.

We can be healed! We can be free from the life-long agonies and heavy loads which we have carried. We can be free from rejection and fear. We can be free to enjoy our relationships with others. We can be free! WE CAN BE FREE!

DELIVERANCE

CHAPTER 6

Deliverance, a scary, controversial word. It conjures up scenes from the movie, the Exorcist, full of violence and insanity. Is deliverance a valid form of healing in today's Christianity? Do Christians even need to be concerned about fighting an invisible entrenched enemy? As "Don", a forty year old executive remarked, "I'm a Christian. How can satan and Jesus dwell in the same place? Christians can't be possessed."

"Sarah", his wife, scoffed, "As if anyone can be possessed. I think that philosophy is pretty archaic, you know, like from the Dark Ages. It seems like when you start talking about the devil, you're getting into the area of witch hunting, looking for a demon under every rock. Isn't that a little far-fetched?"

Good questions. Louis and Carol are asked those questions as well as others as they minister across the country. The answer begins with Ephesians 6:12.

"For our struggle is not against flesh and blood, but against the rulers, against the authorities, against the powers of this dark world and against the spiritual forces of evil in the heavenly realms." (NIV)

Satan and his cohorts are loose in this world. Many of us would love to deny the existence of the evil one. If he did not exist, then it wouldn't be quite so essential to live a life of holiness. We could fudge a little around the edges of our Christian commitment. Denying the magnitude of the spiritual warfare that is going on around us gives a feeling of pseudo-safety. Denial is always dangerous. Denying the presence and the power of the sworn enemy of God is particularly deadly. He moves in for the kill, and we don't even know what hit us. We end up down for the count. According to Hosea 4:6 (NIV), **"my people are destroyed from a lack of knowledge. Because you have rejected knowledge, I also reject you as my priests; because you have ignored the law of your God, I also will ignore your children."** It is critical that we are aware of the demonic activity around us because the lack of knowledge of spiritual warfare can spell defeat, even unto death. This applies to us, our children, and our own child heart. Ignorance of the enemy doesn't make him go away.

That doesn't make witch-hunting a sanctioned holiness sport. A lot of the problems in our lives are caused by old fashioned selfishness; an out-of-control self-life. But, that self-life can open the door to satanic strongholds which, while not possessing Christians, certainly can harass and oppress any believer who allows it to happen.

A person who is satanically possessed has allowed satan to completely control his life. A Christian is one who has given ownership of his life to Jesus. However, because of ignorance of the strength of the self-life and its connections with the demonic, he is still allowing his soul to be in turmoil. Romans 7:15 (NIV) says, **"I do not understand what I do. For what I want to do I do not do, but what I hate I do."** This reflects the struggle common to us all.

Oppression is a recurring harassment of our souls. It enters in our lives through an open door of sin. Even our reactions to the sins committed by others against us can allow the door of oppression to open. There is a relationship between sin and the demonic. Where the former is present, the latter is not far away.

"Alex" would blow up at the slightest provocation. Knowing the principles of spiritual warfare, he tried to bind the spirit of anger.

"In the name of Jesus, I bind this spirit of anger that has been harassing me all of my life. I cut it off at its roots. It will not bother me anymore. Lord, I ask that you fill that gap with your Holy Peace. Thank you Father that you have given me this ability through the power of Your Blood. Amen."

Alex would do really well for a couple of weeks, but soon he would begin to have problems getting angry once again. His temper would really flare after a conversation with his father who also had trouble with anger.

As he received ministry, it became apparent that Alex had never forgiven his father for all of the times his dad had yelled and stormed at him when Alex was a kid. Not only did he have unforgiveness towards his father but he also had some bitterness which had developed from sitting in judgment of his dad's behavior. Unforgiveness and bitterness were the open doors in Alex's life which had allowed demonic oppression to enter in his life in the form of anger. Although he would bind it up away from his life in the proper scriptural manner, it would continue to harass him. No matter how hard he would pray, he couldn't get victory. Alex allowed this see-sawing to occur on a spiritual level because the bitterness and unforgiveness kept the door open for the satanic attack to keep coming from him. As soon as he realized this, Alex had to make a decision to forgive his father and repent of judging him. It wasn't easy for him to do. He had carried those feelings with him for a long time. They had become a part of his life. And without a doubt, his father had severely harmed Alex because of his anger. But, Alex still had to let them go. When he was willing to get rid of them, the healing could begin. Then he was able to get release of the anger which had troubled him for so long. During the healing process, when the sin of judgement and unforgiveness was uncovered and dealt with, he was ready for deliverance. Quite often Christians are inexperienced in how to deal with these problem areas and need to seek assistance from mature believers experienced in deliverance prayers. He finally became free of all of the harassment of that oppressing spirit. Permanently.

To answer an earlier question, no, Christians cannot be possessed. They can, however, be oppressed.

There are open doors which allow the oppression to enter in and harass the Christian. As mentioned earlier, in Alex's case it was bitterness and judgment of his father's offenses. Some of the more common are:

Unforgiveness,
Bitterness,
Judgement,
Resentment,
Offense,
Denial (pride is its root),
Stubbornness,
Self-Pity,
Immorality,
Control,
Dishonesty,
Greed,
Soul ties,
Generational.

Quite a list isn't it? It pays to close those doors. Our lives become much more fruitful. To close them, we need to recognize the problem, repent of allowing it in our lives, and forgive ourselves and anyone else who was responsible for its development. Get some prayer agreement and address these different spirits in the name of Jesus and command them to leave and go to dry places. If the problem recurs there may be a need to seek assistance from someone mature enough in ministry to exercise their authority.

Very simple. Very easy. Very calm. Very scriptural. That is the beginning of the process of deliverance in anyone's life.

Even someone with very serious problems can experience a "quiet deliverance". One man had a compulsion with adultery. He was unable to stay faithful to his wife. He couldn't find enough peace of mind to sleep at night. He couldn't concentrate at work. The speed of his downhill plunge was increasing. His deliverance began when Louis gave him a daddy's hug; a hug of unconditional love, forgiveness, and acceptance that he did not receive as a young child from his own father. Subsequent ministry dealt with other problem areas. That night the man was able to sleep through the night for the first time in a year and a half. He was soon reunited with his family. Sounds simplistic? It can be, when the Lord has His way.

There is no need for the violence and demonic manifestations like some people mistakenly believe. It's not necessary. When preceded by forgiveness and repentance, a quiet deliverance takes place. Strongholds are torn down. Peace, relief, and stability bloom.

When we have been deeply hurt, we may think it is impossible to forgive. The Scripture assures us that **"nothing is impossible with God"** (Luke 1:37 NIV). If we will enter into the process of healing, Jesus will gently peel off layer after layer of dead or putrid "emotion cells". Then He will replace it with His resurrection life in our hearts and minds.

When we do things in any area of our lives, either innocently or intentionally, which are against God's plan, we open ourselves to destruction. As children, we are intended to be covered with an umbrella of innocence. Through a sinful, sexual encounter, for example: seeing someone naked, being fondled, walking in on parents having sex, being molested or abused, exposed to pornography, etc., this innocency bubble bursts. This causes sexual perversion spirits, unclean and defiling spirits, and feelings of guilt and unworthiness to be assigned in one degree or another. Once sexual perversion has made its presence known, the child is very likely to encounter further wounding in this area as he grows older. If sexual perversion has already entered the family, a child can be assigned these before birth and then later encounters are even more wounding.

When there is sexual contact before or outside of the marriage covenant, negative soul ties form. Parts of our souls are fragmented out to each of the other people. **"And when Shechem the son of Hamor the Hivite, the prince of the country, saw her, he took her, and lay with her, and defiled her. And his soul clave unto Dinah the daughter of Jacob, and he loved the damsel, and spake kindly unto the damsel."** (Gen. 34:2,3 KJV) **"His own iniquities shall ensnare the wicked, and he shall be held with the cords of his sin."** (Prov. 5:22 AMP) During ministry, we (Louis and Carol) have seen dramatic healing effects take place. Following repentance, we have broken the negative soul ties, cast out the spirit of destruction (Heb. ABADDON), and called back the fragments of the soul. We also speak out a purifying of the person's total being; spirit, soul and body; and ask God for a restoration of innocence by the Blood of Jesus.

In ministering to people, if we (Louis and Carol) find that there is a problem with double-mindedness one more step is added. The oppression is commanded to leave from both sides of the mind. This is very important.

With one couple, the husband, "Bill", was a practicing homosexual. He had tried to go straight, but couldn't. Several psychiatric doctors had finally given up on him. Every time Bill attempted normality, he would fail. He had become so despondent that he was ready to give up. Although in his heart he deeply wanted his life to change, he was prepared to leave his home, divorce his wife in an effort to get away from himself.

After spending several hours ministering to him, the Lord showed Louis that he needed to command the spiritual oppression to leave all of the Bill Smiths!

Why plural? Why both sides of the mind? Satan and the powers of darkness are masters at legal technicalities. They are legalists. When Louis would command the oppression to leave, which Bill had given him permission to do, satan would use Bill's double-mindedness to travel back and forth from one side of the mind to the other, still staying with the person. By commanding out of all of the Bill Smiths, there was no legal loophole in which the powers of darkness could hide. They had to go. Bill received instant healing. His marriage was restored, and he is now in the ministry living completely for the Lord.

"(For the weapons of our warfare are not carnal, but mighty through God to the pulling down of strongholds;) Casting down imaginations, and every high thing that exalteth itself against the knowledge of God, and bringing

into captivity every thought to the obedience of Christ." (II Cor 10:4,5 KJV) Reality is not just what we pick up with our five senses. Reality includes all that pertains to our lives -- spirit, soul, and body. It is the Word of God that will open our eyes to all that is going around us at every level.

"Lou" battled for years with feelings of suicide, almost her entire life. Even after she became a Christian, she occasionally had to struggle with urges of self-destruction. When she heard about the Gordon's ministry, she was very skeptical. But she was also weary of struggling, so she went through the Heart Mender classes and had her wounded child heart healed. She wanted to be totally healed so she asked for the prayer of deliverance concerning the suicidal tendencies. We prayed for her and she hasn't been bothered since.

If one feels deliverance is needed, seek out mature, loving Christians who are anointed to minister. Our experience in deliverance has been that it can be quiet and effectual once the heart is ready. This preparation through forgiveness and repentance is essential.

Those of us with wounded child hearts often need some type of quiet deliverance after the healing process has begun. Before and after deliverance, the person needs to be consistent in regular daily Bible study. As the oppressing spirit is being bound up and its roots cut off from someone's life, we loose the peace of God in their lives. When the harasser decides to come back with seven of his cohorts, they will find the old place totally filled with godliness. They will flee.

Deliverance is very personal. A person must decide for himself if he wants to walk in total freedom or not. We can't choose it for anyone but ourselves. If a loved one is needing some deliverance, pray for them to have their eyes opened to the truth. Never, though, try to deliver someone who is not open to this revelation. Not only is it dangerous, but it is not how the Lord operates. He doesn't push people into areas when they are not ready.

Micah 7:7-9 (AMP) states, **"Rejoice not against me, O my enemy; when I fall, I shall arise; when I sit in darkness, the Lord shall be a light to me. I will bear the indignation of the Lord, because I have sinned against Him, until He pleads my cause and executes judgement for me. He will bring me forth to the light, and I shall behold His righteous deliverance."**

When we do get ready for His Will, He is waiting for us. His desire for us is that we walk in peace and freedom and be at rest. A quiet deliverance will combat the harassment and oppression that has been shadowing our lives and affecting our relationships. Allow the Lord to continue the healing process. Be willing to release the hurts. Close the open doors through forgiveness and repentance. Seek godly anointed help in praying for deliverance. As freedom is gained, be sure to ask God to release His peace to fill up empty spaces. Feed daily on God's Word. Enjoy the victory. Enjoy the peace!

WHEN IT'S YOUR FAMILY

CHAPTER 7

"Lloyd" and "Lois" were heartsick. Their beautiful teen-age daughter "Linda" had gone on a rebellious rampage. She was dating the worst character they had ever seen and was running with the wrong crowd. No matter what her parents did, she was always angry and upset. Not only was she not showing up at her part-time job, but she was regularly ignoring her curfew. Tonight, Linda's boss had called to say that once more she had not come to work. Lloyd had had it.

Before she had barely made it through the front door, he was ready for her. He stormed, "Enough is enough! You have gone too far this time, Linda. I've had all I'm going to take from you. You just thought things were rough, well, from now on we are going to have martial law. You will come straight home from school. From here your mother will drive you directly to work. When you're not at work, you will be in your room studying. Since you won't give up those sleazy friends of yours, you simply won't get an opportunity to see them. Your social life has now come to an end. I will not have you making a spectacle of yourself or our family with your behavior. Oh, and on Sundays, you better be ready for church. I am sick of the way you have been behaving. It's over."

Linda fought back until the entire family was worn out from all of the strife. Every day dawned to a new battle. No one was happy. The problems compounded and hurt feelings grew deeper. It was war. Finally, Linda ran away from home.

For months Lloyd and Lois heard nothing from her. As they worried about her, the pain was so great that they felt like something had died in their hearts.

One evening as they were praying, Linda called them.

"Hello, dad?"

"Linda! Where are you? What have you been doing? Why haven't you called? What do you think you...."

"DAD, Don't start on me. I mean it. I'll hang up" she threatened.

"Okay, okay, Linda, come home."

"Well, I'll need some money to get home. I'm pretty bummed right now, and I don't have any cash to buy a bus ticket. How about it, you want to send me some money?"

"I'll send you a ticket. Just get yourself home."

Her visit lasted all of one stormy week before she took off again. A couple of more months passed before she called, once more asking for money to get home. And once more conflict caused her visit to last just a week before she flipped out under the pressure, and she headed out of town.

Weary, from the yo-yo emotional tirades, Lloyd and Lois bottomed out in a heap of hopelessness. They just couldn't handle the situation any more, it was getting worse, not better. They finally completely turned their load over to the Lord.

As they sought Him in desperation for wisdom and healing, they began to receive the revelation of the child heart teaching for their own lives. Realizing that the teaching was for them, they received healing for their fractured, bitter hearts. For the first time in years, they knew peace.

They began to examine their relationship with their daughter and began to pray over the condition of her child heart. They discovered that, like them, she too probably had a wounded child heart. Her wounding had occurred as Lloyd was building his business right after she was born. He had worked every waking hour developing a construction company, while Lois had to spend all of her time doing the books and answering the phones. Little Linda was very low on the priority list. Later, when the work load lightened, Linda was in school, busy with activities. So, Lloyd and Lois still did not spend much quality or quantity time with her. Linda grew up always feeling unimportant where her family was concerned. Rejection in a wounded child heart will erupt as rebellion as the child grows older. Linda spent every fiber of her being in rebellion as she grew up.

Learning that the root of Linda's problems were caused from a wounded child heart, Lloyd and Lois sought the Lord for guidance on how to handle the situation. They already knew that anger did not work. Tough love drove her further from them, and laying down the law caused her to run away to the other side of the country. Everything they had done in their own power and knowledge had failed. They knew that in order for her to get well and have peace, they would have to have God's help in developing and restoring a relationship with their daughter. Lloyd and Lois looked past Linda's behaviors and saw the rejection and pain in her wounded child heart. One evening, at peace with one another and with the Lord, and with whole, complete child hearts, they were able to pray quietly, knowing that they could rest upon the Lord to handle any situation. A deep, unconditional love welled up within them for Linda. They felt the Heavenly Father's type of love for their daughter. A love that was so strong they knew they would love her no matter what she did. They felt a real power in that agape love as it became a reality while they were praying for her. Then they began to pray the price. The Lord showed Lloyd his mistakes. He revealed that Lloyd had great anger towards his daughter. Lloyd also harbored unforgiveness and bitterness towards her because of her lifestyle and her rebellion. Immediately, Lloyd repented for judging his daughter. He also repented unto the Lord about the mistakes he had made with Linda. Then Lloyd and Lois forgave Linda for all of the hurtful, shameful acts she had committed.

After asking forgiveness from the Lord for themselves and then forgiving their daughter, they asked Him to reveal to them what oppressing spirits were tormenting their daughter. They bound them up and loosed the power of the Heavenly Father over her life. Lloyd and Lois also began praying the Word over her.

Soon after, Linda called home, extremely hostile. Harshly, she told her parents that she wasn't going to come home. Lloyd and Lois calmly replied, "We love you, Linda. Let us know when you are ready."

Her hostility cooled at their acceptance of her, and they were able to have a civil conversation.

The Lord had shown Lloyd and Lois not to set a time frame in the healing process for Linda. Their decision to allow her to change at her speed rather than theirs took a great deal of pressure off the situation.

For forty days and nights Lloyd and Lois prayed for their daughter. Instead of looking at the near hopeless circumstances, they confessed the Word over her life. They began to see her in a new light based upon the Scriptures. Because their own child hearts were healing, they were able to trust the Lord to take care of bringing her home safely. Lloyd and Lois' prayers were bearing fruit. Linda was soon calling home on a regular basis, sometimes just to chat.

After over a month had passed, the doorbell rang late one night. Lloyd and Lois ran to the door with hope in their hearts. Eagerly unlocking the door, they saw Linda standing on the doorstep. Just like the father of the prodigal son, they welcomed her with open arms.

Linda did not leave again. The war was over. But, there were still spiritual skirmishes that had to be worked out, however. It was as if Linda was going to push them to the limits of their unconditional love to see if they really would continue in it towards her. She had never experienced anything like it and wanted to see if it was genuine. Lloyd and Lois did not waver. They were able to walk in that deep agape love because they continued in heavy-duty prayer, often several hours at a time. They were determined to see total victory.

Finally, Linda came to them in tears.

"Daddy," Linda choked with emotion said, "Help me, Daddy, help me to become a Christian. I'm ready to get serious about getting my life together. I'm ready for whatever you have in your life." The family spent the most joyful evening they ever had together.

Today, several years after that decisive night, Linda is still walking with the Lord. She and her new husband attend church with her parents. Their times together are times of laughter and good fellowship. All deeply love each other with whole, healed hearts and give all of the glory to the Lord. With Him all things are possible.

It is an out and out lie that your children, parents, or spouse will never change. Jesus is MORE than able to minister to them in the spirit as we pray for them and enter into uncompromising spiritual warfare on their behalf. To recover a loved one from the grasp of the enemy, apply the following principles to your situation.

1. Seek healing for your own wounded child heart.
2. Repent. (Yes, there's that word again!)
   Repent of any anger and judgment you have held against that person.

3. Forgive. (Yes, this word is here also.)
   Forgive that individual for their actions and attitudes which have embarrassed you or even harmed you.
4. Come against specific oppressions.
   In the name of Jesus bind up the enemies' strongholds as the Lord reveals them to you. Break their power and cancel their assignments and effects against "all the Bill Smiths" (because of to double-mindedness). Do this on a daily basis until the demonic darkness lifts from their minds. Agree that the Holy Spirit ministers light to their deep needs.
5. Loose the peace and power of God.
   Ask God to loose his wonderful peace and might power over the situation.
6. Pray the Word.
   Pray the Word over your loved one. Claim God's specific promises. Establish a faith vision based upon the Word. See the loved one as he or she can be in the Spirit, beyond the circumstances.
7. Rest and rejoice in God's Ability.
   Continue to trust Him. Praise Him. Often times, those who praised, led the army into battle, defeating the enemy.

This is not deliverance. As mentioned in an earlier chapter, deliverance is to be done with someone who is ready and willing to rid himself of spiritual oppressions. Battling the enemy for a loved one, which family members (particularly parents and spouses) have authority to do, is not deliverance. It is binding up the oppressions so that the individual can begin to make free choices. Deliverance is prayer with the person to rid him of the enemy's oppression.

Lloyd and Lois discovered victory by working through those steps. Their story is not an unusual one in any respect, either. As parents with wounded child hearts, it is very likely that we have passed down pain and rejection to the next generation, and our children probably also have some degree of a wounded child heart. Observe them. When pressure and stress come against them, they will act out, often in an unacceptable manner; usually in rebellion, anger, and hurt. It's tough for a Christian parent to come against this, especially when television and peers reinforce these behaviors. In looking at a critically serious problem, we see the occult is growing with new teenage members every day by fostering and encouraging all "feel-good" destructive attitudes and behaviors. Satanism gives a sense of belonging, acceptance and personal power by feeding the aches of the wounded child heart in our children. A satanist will look for those who are walking in pain because he knows that those are the most susceptible to pseudo-acceptance.

Our children can be reached for God. They, like Linda, can receive healing. As parents, we need to step out. We need to:

1. Nurture the child with the Word.
2. Cover him in prayer.
3. Teach the child to respond correctly to authority and to honor authority.

4. Correct in love, and,
5. Begin to love the child genuinely and unconditionally.

Other members of our families can also be reached. If it is a husband who has the wounded child heart, pray I Timothy 3:2-13 over him, inserting his name in the appropriate places. Respect his position in the household. Continue to show him unconditional love. There will be changes in the marriage relationship if even just one of the partners receives healing of the child heart. It alters the dynamic of all marital interaction.

The same goes for a wife who has a fractured, defensive child heart. The healed husband should pray the Word. He should use Proverbs 31:10-31 for starters. A husband can help bring huge changes by giving his wife unconditional love. That type of love changes things rapidly. The secret is to continue in it. Don't give up when the spouse's behavior deteriorates. That is usually a testing, a proving time, to see if you really mean that kind of deep love. Stand fast.

It is also a temptation to stop praying or acting in love after a change for the better! We do not change at God's direction in order to make someone else change! That's manipulation and deception! Walking in acceptance and love is the LIFESTYLE of a believer! This is required of us every day of our lives until Jesus takes us home!

Dealing with parents can be the most difficult of all. Even if they really seem set in their attitudes, they are still the parents, and see you as a child no matter what the age. Again, as with other relationships where there needs to be healing, pray the Word. Love unconditionally. See beyond the circumstances and the memories and view them as the Lord does: precious. Be sure to forgive. It's very likely that they played a big role in your feelings of rejection. Understand that they were living a script that their parents and circumstances handed them. They probably did not know any better. Be compassionate towards your parents. More than likely, they hate their mistakes which caused you rejection and pain. On the other hand, they may deny any responsibility. Allow the Holy Spirit to deal with this--don't be tempted to bring "correction" yourself.

We need to plant good seed for our family's healing. The Word teaches the principle of sowing and reaping. We sow seed, then we get back a harvest of the same. As we sow into the Spirit, we can trust the Father to bring in the harvest and bless us. But, when we sow things of the enemy, then that's the kind of harvest reaped.

Some Christians begin with great enthusiasm to sow in the Spirit, speak the Word, and stand in faith. The enemy then starts up his whispering campaign to get them off track. "Panic. Do it yourself. It's a critical situation. Hurry. It's a matter of life and death." Anxiety sets in. We'll try to help God out by doing things in the natural all by ourselves. Or maybe we'll push and shove to make things happen. This is manipulation and is a perversion of the sowing and reaping principle.

Reach into the spirit realm by praying, acting on the Word, and trusting the Lord to bring the harvest of those things which we have prayed and spoken. Thank God, He is faithful, and brings His Word to pass. Praise the Lord that we are able to do what it says in the Word for us to do in order to have all needs met. It doesn't matter how bleak it looks in the natural. (And for some of us it has looked pretty bleak!) It doesn't even matter if it looks like it will work out or not. That's not important. God honors our obedience in following His Word. He will bring victory.

When we pray about something, we need to believe that it is answered. Mark 11:23-24 (NIV) says, **"I tell you the truth, if anyone says to this mountain, 'Go, throw yourself into the sea,' and does not doubt in his heart but believes that what he says will happen, it will be done for him. Therefore, I tell you, whatever you ask for in prayer, believe that you have received it and it will be yours."**

A quick test to check to see if we are really believing:

1. We no longer need to worry.
2. We become single-minded.
3. We think, talk, and act differently, and,
4. We praise God for the answer ahead of time.

Then we will see some answers.

Most of us have to deal with a relative whose bizarre, even hateful, behavior drives us right up the wall. But, we have to decide. Are we going to play the part of the devil by accusing them or are we going to act as God wants us to? There is absolutely no middle ground, none at all.

Matthew 6:24 (Amp) reminds us, **"No man can serve two masters; for either he will hate the one and love the other, or he will stand by and be devoted to the one and despise and be against the other. You cannot serve God and mammon (that is, deceitful riches, money, possessions,**

or what is trusted in)." We cannot trust what the carnal mind feeds us about the circumstances and truly trust God at the same time. The circumstances are not the "facts", they are subject to change. What God says about the person or situation is what is true. When we speak in agreement with the rhema word about these circumstances, God's Word, and faith in His Word, will move mountains.

As we seek guidance from the Lord, the Holy Spirit will show us how to pray for loved ones, how to bind the demonic activity of the powers of darkness. The answers the Lord gives will always bless us.

In walking out His directions, the flesh will always go the direction the mind goes. When the soul lines up with the Word of God, the body will also line up. If the mind is reprobate, so will the flesh be. There is great power in the mind, will and emotions, but it is subservient to godly authority. The true authority is only in the Spirit. Power and authority come when spirit and soul are aligned with God and when that happens, there will be amazing strength in the Christian walk. Your home will become a peaceable haven.

There are areas in every family which have been fought over for so long and in so many ways, that they have become red flag subjects. Offense has taken root and flourished. Rather than fight anymore, communication is eventually shut down. No one talks about the problems. They become closed subjects. Satan uses these "hot potato" topics as entryways into the life of the family.

It can be about money, family problems, friendships, other relatives, hobbies, politics, many things. Those who have experienced red flag areas know exactly how quickly temperatures can rise over the introduction of those volatile subjects. How is it possible to get around this mess?

Again, unconditional love is the door for healing to flow through. To communicate, we need to lay down our highmindedness and walk in love. Go to that family member and humbly say, "My perception may be wrong, but I believe that we have a problem in this area and I value your input. I would like to hear how this looks to you. Then, let's pray and hear from God."

When we come together humbly, quietly, peaceably and in love to discuss even the toughest of things, peace will enter our lives and our hearts.

Our loved ones can know that healing. They can know peace. They can have healthy, happy, and whole child hearts. Territory can be retaken. Don't allow any family member to slip away. Reclaim them. Be willing to learn how to gently communicate. Be willing to look past the circumstances. Be willing to be wrong. Be willing to pray the price and receive victory. Allow the Lord to lead you into a new dimension of love for your family and enjoy your new relationships.

A WHOLE AND COMPLETE LIFE

CHAPTER 8

"Arise, shine; for thy light is come, and the glory of the Lord is risen upon thee. For, behold, the darkness shall cover the earth, and gross darkness the people: but the Lord shall arise upon thee, and his glory shall be seen upon thee." (Isa. 60:1,2 KJV) **"The people that have walked in darkness have seen a great light: they that dwell in the land of the shadow of death, upon them hath the light shined."** (Isa. 9:2 KJV)

As the light of God's Word begins to shine in our hearts, more and more freedom will come. As we begin to experience the healing of our child hearts, ask the Lord to send prayer support. We should begin to pray more. Sing worship and praise to God from the heart. If this is something new, playing praise music will help.

A few warnings will be helpful. First of all, the enemy of our souls is not going to be pleased that there is healing going on! He will attack the mind in familiar areas. All kinds of fearful thoughts will be sent to harass. Stay in the Word so that there will be ammunition to fire back! "NO, DEVIL! I'M NOT BUYING YOUR LIES ANY MORE! GOD'S WORD SAYS...."! (That is exactly how Jesus showed us to deal with those temptations in Matthew 4 and Luke 3.) Whether the lie is rejection, confrontation, abandonment, losing control, physical pain, or poverty, WE DON'T HAVE TO ACT ON IT ANYMORE! The Lord is standing right beside us to back up His Word when we speak it! **"I have set the LORD always before me. Because he is at my right hand, I will not be shaken."** (Psalm 16:8 NIV) God has provided freedom and healing for us at the Cross of Calvary. Jesus did the work to heal and cleanse us completely and totally.

While we walk in the freshness of our healing, the enemy will try to replay all the old things that were in our souls. He will try to chain us again into all of those old life patterns. The trumpet of hope sounds in triumph as we recognize those things in our lives which do not reflect what the Lord says and teaches. Rather than feeling condemned about that old baggage, we can reach towards the Lord, knowing He is more than able to heal. The Lord has forgiven us of our sins, all of them, no matter what they have been.

Our problem is that we usually haven't allowed Jesus to be Redeemer in all of the areas in our lives. As previously stated, it could have been shame or even denial. It could even have been a lack of faith that kept Jesus at bay; that kept Him from entering the dark hidden closets of our hearts. Until Jesus is received as Redeemer in a specific area and Healer in a specific area, the enemy blitzes our minds with bombs of guilt, confusion, and turmoil. God does not torment us with memories. When He brings something to light, it is radiant with healing.

It is the enemy who keeps records of our sins. The Lord erases the memory of the junkyards of our sins from His presence through the precious Blood of Jesus. Accepting the cleansing power of the Blood makes our lives whole. If we continue to allow satan to condemn and berate us about former hurtful, even shameful areas, we are not letting Jesus be Lord over those areas. We take them back, jerking bits and pieces of our lives out of the loving hands of the Father, opening our lives up to failure.

We know now, that we can be healed. We no longer have to buy into satan's lies which dictate certain actions and attitudes to make ourselves feel okay. We can be healed of destructive behaviors.

God can and will bring life to that which is dead. He breaks the concrete in which the devil had mired us. We do not have to stay in the old position. The Lord pulls us out of the miry pit and places us on the Rock. He desires to put a song of praise in our hearts each and every day.

Positionally, we have been free since we received Jesus as Savior, but we have to daily walk trusting Him to experience the freedom of this grace. **"So, my dear friends, just as you have always obeyed when I was with you, it is even more important that you obey now when I am away from you: keep working out your deliverance with fear and trembling, for God is the one working among you both the**

willing and the working for what pleases him." (Phil. 2:12,13 JNT) Psalm 130:3,4 (KJV) also reassures us, **"If thou, Lord, shouldest mark iniquities, O Lord, who shall stand? But there is forgiveness with thee, that thou mayest be feared."**

Just reading the newspaper illustrates the amount of destruction which is rampant in the world. The statistics are staggering. Drug abuse, alcoholism, rebellion, divorce, suicide, all race through communities everywhere. Suffering trauma through the process of living, there are multitudes of crippled child hearts. Over and over, generations have been terribly wounded, so that our society has become more and more fragmented and more and more angry. Practically every person alive today carries some type of "battle scars". But, because of Jesus, none of us has to stay burdened by them. Because He is God, He has the ability to spend the time to work with each one all the time to heal and to cleanse.

One illustration of the healing process should be recognized. As we take secret hurts and rejections to the Lord for healing, a purging occurs. From the depths of our hearts, this cleansing scrubs away the ugliness and strips away the scarring.

When a small child falls on gravel, his little knees really hurt. Gravel burns are some of the most hurtful little injuries. If left alone, particles of rock and small pieces of dirt fester. The memories of the accident are underscored by continual pain because the knee hasn't been cleaned. There might be infection or swelling. The trusty bandage won't even help.

Cleaning out the little knee will not only be just a little uncomfortable, but the actual purging of the dirt and gravel can even be quite painful. But it is a different, quicker, healing type of hurt. And then it is over, the little knee gets well. The small child quickly gets back to the business of life. All is well. All is secure.

All can be well and secure for us, too. Jesus provides wholeness. Jesus is our security. He shows us how to really live. He promised that when He ascended to the right hand of the Father, that He would send the Holy Spirit to be in us and to comfort us. He even said, (John 16: 7,13a NIV), **"But I tell you the truth: It is for your good that I am going away. Unless I go away, the Counselor will not come to you; but if I go, I will send him to you...But when he, the Spirit of truth, comes, he will guide you into all truth."**

Some of the symbols of the Holy Spirit in the Bible are wind, fire, water, and oil. In the healing of child heart hurts, we can recognize His rhythms. The wind of the Spirit fills the bellows which stir up the fire under the crucible of our daily lives. As the fire burns hotter the sediment of old hurts comes to the surface to be washed away by the purifying, cleansing water of the Spirit. Then the oil comes in to sooth and heal. This same oil begins to soften the next layer of sludge, so that as the wind again begins to blow, more sediment is able to be brought to the surface. This process of the loving hand of God continues to cleanse and purify us.

We can grow in confidence that Jesus will not leave or forsake us, that He has us safely in His embrace, that He loves us. Our self life will not need defending any more.

We no longer have to be perfect all of the time. We can be secure in the safety of His love, the way we were created to be.

"And eternal life is this: to know You, the one true God, and Him Whom You sent, Yeshua the Messiah" (John 17:3 JNT). So, the Lord not only desires us to be healthy and whole in all circumstances, He provides the way.

When the heart has been wounded, the child within needs to be made whole, accepted, and loved. When the heart is healed, there is joy, a settled peaceable child heart, singleness of mind and heart, trusting God rather than in their emotions, personal strength, intellect, or circumstances.

Let's follow His path. Let's walk in His healing. Let's destroy the defense mechanisms which have been ruling in our lives at the root. Let's begin forgiving those who have hurt us and repent of having judged them. Let us walk in the fullness of our Christianity unafraid to push back traditional boundaries, and bask in His unconditional love. Let's walk in victory with a healed, whole child heart. It's possible. Enjoy the new life Jesus provides.

It is not difficult for Him to reign in our circumstances; what causes Him difficulty is the withholding of our hearts from Him! If there has been lots of destruction in our lives, His promise is restoration. **"And I will restore to you the years that the locust hath eaten, the cankerworm, and the caterpillar, and the palmerworm, my great army which I sent among you. And ye shall eat in plenty, and be satisfied, and praise the name of the Lord your God, that hath dealt wondrously with you: and my people shall never be ashamed."** (Joel 2:25-26 KJV)

By the choices that we make, we can bear much fruit for the Kingdom of God, or we can go down into defeat by agreeing with the works of darkness. Gal. 5:22-23 (KJV) says that **"the fruit of the Spirit is love, joy, peace, longsuffering, gentleness, goodness, faith, meekness, temperance:"** If we want to allow the Holy Spirit to produce this fruit then we need to continually search the Word. The Word will wash our thought life and enable us to adopt new attitudes.

Oh, beloved! Don't resist the purifying work of the Holy Spirit! This is the means by which we are transformed into His image!

TESTIMONIES

The biggest immediate change that I noticed after my initial "Mommy and Daddy hug" was that the little girl inside of me quit crying. It was "the beginning" of "a process of getting to a place of emotional healing". I learned that the wound in my child heart was the doorway (i.e. entry point) for demonic activity to manifest through me. It prevented me from being able to possess my own soul, as Jesus commands us to do. (Luke 21:19 KJV) Until I began to experience healing and deliverance, I was unable to control or even express my emotions in a way that did not wound myself or others.

I am so thankful and grateful for all that God has done to set me free, and I know there is more to come. **-D.**

One of the things the Lord revealed during child heart ministry was an early childhood experience. At the age of three, I recalled my mother leaving me to go on a trip to my grandmother's. They stayed for several days. She took my older brother and younger sister, but left me at home with a teenage babysitter.

As they drove away, I remember how upset, hurt, and fearful I was. Was I bad? Or not good enough or what? My "seemingly innocent" responses caused me to accept rejection, resentment, judgement, unforgiveness, etc. Year after year, as those sins stayed in place, I built on that foundation. Not until I learned to repent and forgive could I be set free from years of pain.

This demonstrates how very small children (sometimes even before remembrance) can open the doors or be attacked by sin. **-G.**

The teaching and ministry I received from the Lord through Louis and Carol concerning the child heart has totally transformed my life!

The inability to "live up to my potential" as my grade school teachers put it, insecurities in dating in high school, problems with my parents, getting in trouble with the law, wanting to succeed at college but failing, the failure at one job or business venture after another, turning to alcohol, drugs, pornography, "singles" bars and promiscuity, anything to try to satisfy that inner longing to be accepted, to quit hurting, to feel loved, but always coming up short, all stemmed from the wounded child heart.

Over the years, this double-mindedness caused by deep-seated hidden insecurity, hurt, betrayal, and rejection on one hand, with pride, rebellion, worldliness and fear on the other, led me to deep inner rage, despair, financial bondage, and the breakup of a marriage that began in a Bible-believing church.

When I got married, my spouse and I didn't understand much of anything spiritually, especially about why we felt the way we did inside, and did the things we did. Our church didn't have any kind of ministry in this area, so gradually, we slid into the same old life patterns, not knowing what was happening and why, and feeling powerless to do anything about it. Life became a struggle to just keep going from one day to the next.

Then, after a personal tragedy several years ago, I came face to face with the reality of the magnitude of failure in every area of my life, admitted to myself just how wounded and miserable inside that I really was, and responded to the call of God and surrendered my heart and life to the Lord Jesus.

It was during this time of total brokenness before the Lord, that I began to see my life from His point of view. I met Louis and Carol through a Bible study group, and began to listen to their tapes, and received some personal ministry from them at one of their seminars. When they gave me a "Mommy and Daddy's hug", and ministered healing to my child heart for the hurt and wounds caused by the inability of my natural parents to truly show me unconditional love, I broke down and wept for hours. Finally, I now could receive the inner peace, comfort, and love that the Lord intended me to have. Within days, my attitudes and behaviors changed drastically.

I began to understand how my reactions to circumstances in life were based upon the set of "instructions" that were stored inside my soul and heart, which came directly from the wounded child heart, and saw how this had adversely affected me all of my life, even though these childhood hurts were not consciously remembered.

After getting free of the bondage that had shaped my life, one of the first things I had to do, was to forgive my parents for the lack of proper nurturing and the hurt I received from them. Next, I had to repent to God for judging them, and I also repented directly to my parents and asked their forgiveness for my rebellion, anger, and the hurt that I had caused them. This was not easy, since this relationship had been lousy for years, and they were not aware of spiritual things, including the child heart.

Although this humbling before God and my parents was difficult, it was absolutely worth it. Since I made the decision to "honor my father and mother", my "days have been long upon the land which the Lord has given me." We have a totally new relationship! We are able to communicate about life, and can give and receive unconditional love to each other for the first time in our lives. We have finally become a true blessing to each other, as the Lord intended. It's never too late.

Over a period of time, as I was faithful to yield to the work of the Holy Spirit in healing and purging my heart from these hurts, my circumstances in life have drastically changed. I am single-minded to serve the Lord Jesus, and no longer feel the craving for drugs, alcohol, or adultery. The obsessive/compulsive behaviors are gone! These behaviors were only the symptoms, not the disease itself. The Lord has directed my life, blessed me, and provided everything I need. I am now able to love and be loved, to trust instead of expecting betrayal, to minister to others, am successful in business and personal endeavors, and know that I have a wonderful future planned by the Lord.

All of this would not have been possible without receiving the teaching and healing found in this book. I pray that anyone who reads this testimony will understand how important this truth about the child heart is, and receives the healing that Jesus wants you to have, too. -S.

A business man in a roller-coaster lifestyle, I was born again, but backslidden. I had allowed alcohol, drugs, and adultery to rule my life. I resisted meeting Louis and Carol, but after I received the hug, I was won over. Prayers of emotional healing and quiet deliverance followed, and my life was changed from darkness to light. Recommitted to Christ, my feet are now on higher ground. **-T.**

As **T.**'s wife, during the thirteen years of trauma, through the pits of hell, I hung on to my family through prayer and spiritual warfare. I had the support of loving, prayerful friends. Louis and Carol have ministered to me and my whole family. We are now able to stand strong and are bringing our lives into order through Jesus.

The healing of the wounded child heart in our lives was a crucial piece of life's puzzle that had been missing. We had been to all kinds of counselors, therapy, etc. to very little avail, until the child heart ministry began in our lives. We are now able to minister more love to our children.
-Mrs. T.

For more information, contact:

Heart Menders
P.O. Box 516
Bethany, OK 73008-0516
(405) 787-3572

We are a teaching and healing ministry. We hold seminars at our home church, Faith Fellowship, 900 N. May, Oklahoma City, OK, on a regular basis. We are available to minister at other churches as the Lord leads.

Tapes and seminars are available on:

The healing of the child heart
Marriage and family healing
Growth in the Spirit
Spiritual warfare for families

There is also a booklet for beginners in the Christian life called "Body Basics, Spiritual Fitness for the Believer". It is excellent for handouts to new converts or for a Sunday school class.

THE FOLLOWING PAGES ARE OUR 1992

RESOURCE CATALOG

<u>SINGLE TAPES</u> <u>$5.00</u>

HM008 WIN THEM TO JESUS
Effective witnessing
HM009 IDOLATRY
Dealing with the hidden idols in your life
HM011 INTIMACYIN MARRIAGE
How to develop intimacy
HM012 FRUIT OF SINGLE-MINDEDNESS
Testimony and teaching
HM020 GIVING AND RECEIVING
Dynamics of Godly interactions
HM021 SOWING AND REAPING
Effecting changes in relationships
HM040 SAFE PLACES
An atmosphere for healing
HM041 HONORING YOUR PARENTS
Family healing
HM043 NOT SO GREAT EXPECTATIONS
Performance orientation
HM044 THE THREE TEMPTATIONS
A look at basics
HM045 JUSTIFYING OURSELVES
How we see ourselves
HM046 POWER OF FORGIVENESS
Basic steps in healing
HM047 PURPOSE FOR YOUR LIFE
God's plan
HM048 YOU <u>CAN</u> DO SOMETHING
Initiating change
HM049 TIGHT PLACES
Under pressure?
HM050 ESTEEM AS PRECIOUS
What do we value?
HM051 CHALLENGE TO CHANGE
Not resisting growth
HM5011 THE TEST
Forgiving yourself
HM6022 THE GONG SHOW
A real love walk

TWO TAPE SERIES **$10.00**

HM202 PREPARING THE HEART
Forgiveness and the traps of the enemy
HM205 LEVIATHAN, PRIDE AND THE SELF-LIFE
The strength of the self exposed
HM206 BREAKING THE STRONGHOLDS OF THE MIND Renewing the mind with scripture
HM207 PRAYER
Improving your prayer life
HM208 TWO-EDGED SWORD
Life changing weapons
HM209 WHO DO YOU TRUST?
Choices about trust

THREE TAPE SERIES **$15.00**

HM301 CHILD HEART HEALING
Healing your child heart
HM302 HOW TO LOVE YOUR HUSBAND
Praying for your spouse
HM303 "...EVEN AS YOUR SOULS PROSPER"
How to deal with your self life
HM304 THE FINE TUNING OF MARRIAGE
From a Nova Shalom seminar
HM305 HOW TO BE AN OVERCOMER
Training the soul to bow to the Spirit
HM306 HOW TO LOVE YOUR WIFE
What the Lord has taught Louis
HM307 AUTHORITY STRUCTURES
God's Plan vs. the Babylonian pattern
HM308 FREEDOM FROM JUDGMENT
Who are we judging?
HM309 BASIC RELATIONSHIP BUILDING
Communication, Sex and Money

FIVETAPESERIES **$25.00**

HM501 DARKNESS AND LIGHT
Uncovering strongholds of darkness and defeating them with the Word

SIX TAPE SERIES **$30.00**

HM601 BUILDINGON THE ROCK
Basic series on dealing with sins of the heart and other foundational principles

HM602 RELATIONSHIP DYNAMICS
Recognising co-dependency, performance orientation, perfectionism, pressure, denial, etc.

HM603 COVENANT LIFE
A basic series on walking out a covenant relationship

HM604 MANHOOD AND WOMANHOOD
How God designed men and women to interact and be blessed by their uniqueness

HM605 SPIRITUAL WARFARE
Preparing for and conducting effective warfare

TEN TAPE SERIES **$50.00**

HM1000 DESIGN FOR MARRIAGE
A rich series dealing with the deep issues which must be dealt with in continued marriage healing. Becoming one, overcoming self-centeredness, dealing with bitterness, familiarity, and offenses. Encouragement in walking through the purifying fire of God.

BOOKS AND BOOKLETS

(Prices includes First Class postage and handling)

THE CHILD HEART	**$9.95**
Louis & Carol Gordon (Price change reflects 1st Class Postage)	
BODY BASICS	**$3.50**
Louis & Carol Gordon	
ALTERNATIVE TO DIVORCE	**$2.75**
Marilyn Conrad	
FIRST AID FOR A WOUNDED MARRIAGE	**$2.75**
Marilyn Phillipps	

HEART MENDERS, INC.
P. O. BOX 516
BETHANY, OK 73008-0516

(405) 787-3572

Mail to:

HEART MENDERS. INC.
P.O. BOX 516
Bethany, OK 73008-0516

Name ______________________________
Address ____________________________
City ______________________________
State ____________________ Zip ____________

Quantity	Item	Cost
TOTAL		
Postage & Handling (See below)		
GRAND TOTAL		

International Orders, Please Send USA Funds

Tape Orders:
Please add $.25 per tape plus $2.00 for Shipping and Handling (Increase reflects First Class mailing costs)

Book Orders:
First Class postage included in book price

OKLAHOMA RESIDENTS, PLEASE ADD SALES TAX